Atlas of Minimally Invasive and Robotic Esophagectomy

Min P. Kim

Editor

Atlas of Minimally Invasive and Robotic Esophagectomy

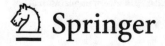 Springer

Editor
Min P. Kim
Division of Thoracic Surgery
Department of Surgery and Cardiothoracic Surgery
Weill Cornell Medical College Department of Surgery
Houston Methodist Hospital
Houston, TX
USA

ISBN 978-3-030-55671-6   ISBN 978-3-030-55669-3   (eBook)
https://doi.org/10.1007/978-3-030-55669-3

This Springer imprint is published by the registered company Springer Nature Switzerland AG
The registered company address is: Gewerbestrasse 11, 6330 Cham, Switzerland

To my wife, Maria, for her love and support.
To my children, Sophia and Alexander, my life's blessing.
To all my patients I had the privilege to serve.

Preface

Surgical treatment of patients with esophageal cancer has evolved. The standard operations for esophageal cancer have been an open procedure where esophageal cancer is resected and an anastomosis is made between gastric conduit to the native esophagus in the chest or the neck. The advancement of minimally invasive instruments provides a new era where we can perform the same operation with smaller incisions that provide fewer morbidity and faster recovery.

The following chapters demonstrate the step-by-step method of performing minimally invasive esophagectomy and robot-assisted esophagectomy. The chapters cover the techniques of performing minimally invasive and robot-assisted Ivor Lewis esophagectomy and McKeown esophagectomy as well as variation in methods of chest and neck anastomosis and a method to perform jejunostomy.

Each author provides a narrative on their technique in performing the esophagectomy with pearls for different parts of the operation. As with any other surgical procedure, there are controversies about how to handle different parts of the operation. Since the goal of the book is not to debate the best method but to provide a method to perform the complex operation in a minimally invasive way, we have kept each author's narrative and viewpoints within the chapter.

This is one of the first Atlas that incorporates robot-assisted esophagectomy techniques. We hope that specialists and trainees will benefit from this Atlas to help treat patients with esophageal cancer.

New York, NY, USA   Min P. Kim
Houston, TX, USA

Contents

Contributors

Shanda H. Blackmon, MD, MPH Department of Surgery, Mayo Clinic Thoracic Surgery, Mayo Clinic Rochester, Rochester, MN, USA

Haydee de Calvo, MD Division of Thoracic Surgery, Department of Surgery, Houston Methodist Hospital, Houston, TX, USA

Edward Y. Chan, MD Department of Surgery and Cardiothoracic Surgery, Weill Cornell Medical College, New York, NY, USA

Division of Thoracic Surgery, Department of Surgery, Houston Methodist Hospital, Houston, TX, USA

Ray Chihara, MD, PhD Department of Surgery and Cardiothoracic Surgery, Weill Cornell Medical College, New York, NY, USA

Division of Thoracic Surgery, Department of Surgery, Houston Methodist Hospital, Houston, TX, USA

Christopher S. Digesu, MD Department of Surgery, Beth Israel Deaconess Medical Center, Harvard Medical School, Boston, MA, USA

Matthew L. Inra, MD Department of Surgery, Mayo Clinic Thoracic Surgery, Mayo Clinic Rochester, Rochester, MN, USA

Department of Cardiothoracic Surgery, Divsion of Thoracic Surgery, Lenox Hill Hospital - Northwell Health, New York, NY, USA

Michael Kent, MD Department of Surgery, Division of Thoracic Surgery and Interventional Pulmonology, Beth Israel Deaconess Medical Center, Harvard Medical School, Boston, MA, USA

Min P. Kim, MD Division of Thoracic Surgery, Department of Surgery and Cardiothoracic Surgery, Weill Cornell Medical College Department of Surgery, Houston Methodist Hospital, Houston, TX, USA

David C. Rice, MB, BCh, BAO, FRCSI Department of Thoracic and Cardiovascular Surgery, Division of Surgery, University of Texas MD Anderson Cancer Center, Houston, TX, USA

Minimally Invasive and Robotic Esophagectomy

Haydee de Calvo and Min P. Kim

Esophageal cancer accounts for about 1% of all new cancer cases. Incidence is highest in males in the sixth to seventh decade of life, with adenocarcinoma being the most common type of esophageal cancer in the United States. Overall, esophageal cancer is a very aggressive type of cancer, with about 20% overall survival at five years after treatment [1]. There is improved survival in patients with an earlier pathologic stage of cancer compared to the later pathologic stage, where surgery plays a vital role in the treatment of esophageal cancer. Multiple studies have shown that a multidisciplinary approach to locally advanced esophageal cancer with surgical resection as an essential part of therapy contributes to survival benefit [2].

Esophagectomy has always been a challenging operation with several different techniques currently practiced in the world. The first esophageal resection for malignancy was performed in 1877 by a Bohemian surgeon named Czerny, but Franz Torek performed the first successful esophagectomy for carcinoma in 1913. Since this time, there has been a succession of modifications and innovative approaches to combat the problematic anatomical location posed when operating on the esophagus. Three standard techniques now include transhiatal, transthoracic, and three-hole approaches. The transhiatal or transabdominal approach requires an abdominal and left neck incision with esophagogastric anastomosis at the level of the left neck. The transthoracic or Ivor Lewis approach uses an abdominal and right chest incision with anastomosis at the level of the right chest. Finally, the three-hole esophagectomy or McKeown esophagectomy includes a right chest, abdomen, and left neck incision with anastomosis at the left neck [3].

A large analysis of the Society of Thoracic Surgeons General Thoracic Surgery Database, including a total of 4321 esophagectomies, shows a perioperative mortality risk of 3.1% and a major comorbidity risk of 33.1%. Within open procedures, the highest mortality risk was identified with Ivor Lewis esophagectomy at 3.8% and the highest morbidity risk at 38.2% for the McKeown esophagectomy [4]. International Japanese Database and national American College of Surgeons National Surgical Quality Improvement Program database analyses have also yielded a similar mortality risk [5, 6]. Recently, Low et al. have developed international consensus definitions for the most common perioperative complications that have provided the community with a common definition of morbidity after esophagectomy [7]. The three most common significant morbidities for esophagectomies are an anastomotic leak, pneumonia, and reintubation [4].

The advent of minimally invasive techniques started with the use of video-assisted thoracoscopy and laparoscopy. At first, hybrid methods were used and found to have promising results. A randomized control trial that compared a hybrid technique of laparoscopy with right thoracotomy vs. total open esophagectomy showed significantly decreased rates of major postoperative morbidity, including pulmonary complications such as acute respiratory distress syndrome and pneumonitis. Overall survival and 30-day mortality were not proven to be significantly different, but there was a trend toward increased overall survival with the hybrid minimally invasive group [8]. In addition, this study, as well as other meta-analysis studies, showed that the minimally invasive esophagectomy group had improved health-care-related quality of life compared to open esophagectomy group [9, 10]. Moreover, minimally invasive esophagectomy does not compromise oncologic resection, which led to an increase in the adoption of minimally invasive esophagectomies [11–13]. Numerous single-center and multicenter studies showed shorter operative times, decreased blood loss, and decreased

H. de Calvo
Division of Thoracic Surgery, Department of Surgery,
Houston Methodist Hospital, Houston, TX, USA

M. P. Kim (✉)
Division of Thoracic Surgery, Department of Surgery and
Cardiothoracic Surgery, Weill Cornell Medical College Department
of Surgery, Houston Methodist Hospital, Houston, TX, USA
e-mail: mpkim@houstonmethodist.org

© Springer Nature Switzerland AG 2021
M. P. Kim (ed.), *Atlas of Minimally Invasive and Robotic Esophagectomy*, https://doi.org/10.1007/978-3-030-55669-3_1

length of intensive care unit stay, and overall hospital length of stay [14–18].

These studies led to the development of the traditional invasive vs. minimally invasive esophagectomy (TIME trial), which was a multicenter, randomized controlled trial in European centers. Straatman et al. found significantly decreased pulmonary infections, blood loss, and hospital stay as well as significantly improved patient-reported outcome measures in the minimally invasive group compared to the traditional group [19]. All of these benefits came without an increase in the anastomotic leak rate, which was the theoretical concern surgeons had with the minimally invasive approach to esophagectomy. Finally, the TIME trial highlighted that the integrity of oncologic resection was not compromised by showing that there were no significant differences in R0 resection rates, lymph node yield, or recurrence rates between minimally invasive and open approaches.

Furthermore, an analysis of the Japanese National Clinical Database, including 24,233 patients, showed mortality and postoperative comorbidity benefit in minimally invasive esophagectomy compared to open approach [20]. As minimally invasive techniques increase in popularity, it is important to note that there is a learning curve to these techniques that can be impactful on the rates of morbidity [21]. This concept becomes crucial as surgeons outside of high-volume centers start adopting minimally invasive methods. Benchmarks have been established from the evaluation of low comorbidity patient groups in the hopes of highlighting this gap and creating a reference point regarding morbidity and mortality rates [22]. As minimally invasive techniques continue to be adopted, we anticipate further data, including the upcoming randomized controlled Randomized Oesophagectomy: Minimally Invasive or Open (ROMIO) trial [23].

When comparing minimally invasive Ivor Lewis vs. McKeown, several studies, including propensity-matched analysis, have shown trends toward decreased rates of mortality and morbidity outcomes with the Ivor Lewis approach [24–26]. Meta-analyses, including over 4000 patients, have identified significantly less recurrent laryngeal nerve injury, blood loss, and length of hospital stay with minimally invasive Ivor Lewis compared to McKeown [27, 28]. Moreover, there was a large population-based study of 3970 patients in the Netherlands that showed increased lymph node yield for a transthoracic esophagectomy approach, whether open or minimally invasive as compared to any transabdominal/transhiatal approach [29]. As mentioned previously, a vital part of esophagectomies is the anastomotic component, as leaks can be detrimental to patient outcomes. Therefore, there have been numerous studies on anastomotic techniques and their associated complications. The results have been varied and controversial. Few studies have shown an increased rate of strictures with hand-sewn anastomosis as compared to stapled [30–32]. Leak rates have also been shown to be increased with hand-sewn anastomosis regardless of anastomotic location, cervical vs. thoracic [31, 33].

As we look to the future of minimally invasive techniques, there has been the incorporation of the robotic systems in esophagectomy. We see the last decade repeating itself as we again try to learn about the robotic system learning curve in the realm of esophagectomies. Two studies have found the need for 70–80 procedures for surgeons to attain a steady level of performance [34, 35]. A randomized controlled trial comparing the robot-assisted minimally invasive esophagectomy to open esophagectomy (ROBOT) showed significantly decreased objective blood loss and cardiopulmonary complications, as well as subjective postoperative pain and improved quality of life scores [36]. When comparing the robotic methods with video-assisted counterparts, the robot has preliminarily been shown to have increased operative time but decreased blood loss and otherwise comparable outcomes [37–40]. With robotic techniques come the advantage of wristed instruments leading to increased dexterity as well as improved visualization into difficult anatomical locations.

Overall, the history of esophagectomies has been rich in changes and particularly in the last decades within the era of technology. As we transitioned from open to hybrid and now totally minimally invasive techniques, we continue to recognize the advantages in morbidity rates. As we continue on the learning curve of technology, we remain focused on extracting the practices that aid us in providing our patients with the best care and continuing to push the limits of clinical science.

References

1. Cancer Stat Facts: Esophageal Cancer: National Cancer Institute. Available from: https://seer.cancer.gov/statfacts/html/esoph.html#survival.
2. Sjoquist KM, Burmeister BH, Smithers BM, Zalcberg JR, Simes RJ, Barbour A, Gebski V. Survival after neoadjuvant chemotherapy or chemoradiotherapy for resectable oesophageal carcinoma: an updated meta-analysis. Lancet Oncol. 2011;12(7):681–92. Epub 2011/06/21. PubMed PMID: 21684205. https://doi.org/10.1016/s1470-2045(11)70142-5.
3. Takahashi C, Shridhar R, Huston J, Meredith K. Esophagectomy from then to now. J Gastrointest Oncol. 2018;9(5):903–9. https://doi.org/10.21037/jgo.2018.08.15. Epub 2018/12/07. PubMed PMID: 30505593; PMCID: PMC6219976.
4. Raymond DP, Seder CW, Wright CD, Magee MJ, Kosinski AS, Cassivi SD, et al. Predictors of major morbidity or mortality after resection for esophageal cancer: a society of thoracic surgeons general thoracic surgery database risk adjustment model. Ann Thorac Surg. 2016;102(1):207–14. https://doi.org/10.1016/j.athoracsur.2016.04.055. Epub 2016/06/01. PubMed PMID: 27240449; PMCID: PMC5016796.
5. Takeuchi H, Miyata H, Gotoh M, Kitagawa Y, Baba H, Kimura W, et al. A risk model for esophagectomy using data of 5354 patients included in a Japanese nationwide web-based database. Ann Surg.

2014;260(2):259–66. Epub 2014/04/20. PubMed PMID: 24743609. https://doi.org/10.1097/sla.0000000000000644.

6. Dhungel B, Diggs BS, Hunter JG, Sheppard BC, Vetto JT, Dolan JP. Patient and peri-operative predictors of morbidity and mortality after esophagectomy: American College of Surgeons National Surgical Quality Improvement Program (ACS-NSQIP), 2005–2008. J Gastrointest Surg. 2010;14(10):1492–501. Epub 2010/09/09. PubMed PMID: 20824375. https://doi.org/10.1007/s11605-010-1328-2.

7. Low DE, Alderson D, Cecconello I, Chang AC, Darling GE, D'Journo XB, et al. International consensus on standardization of data collection for complications associated with esophagectomy: Esophagectomy Complications Consensus Group (ECCG). Ann Surg. 2015;262(2):286–94. Epub 2015/01/22. PubMed PMID: 25607756. https://doi.org/10.1097/SLA.0000000000001098.

8. Mariette C, Markar SR, Dabakuyo-Yonli TS, Meunier B, Pezet D, Collet D, et al. Hybrid minimally invasive esophagectomy for esophageal cancer. N Engl J Med. 2019;380(2):152–62. Epub 2019/01/10. PubMed PMID: 30625052. https://doi.org/10.1056/NEJMoa1805101.

9. Mariette C, Markar S, Dabakuyo-Yonli TS, Meunier B, Pezet D, Collet D, et al. Health-related quality of life following hybrid minimally invasive versus open esophagectomy for patients with esophageal cancer, analysis of a multicenter, open-label, randomized phase III controlled trial: the MIRO Trial. Ann Surg. 2019. Epub 2019/08/14. PubMed PMID: 31404005; https://doi.org/10.1097/SLA.0000000000003559.

10. Kauppila JH, Xie S, Johar A, Markar SR, Lagergren P. Meta-analysis of health-related quality of life after minimally invasive versus open oesophagectomy for oesophageal cancer. Br J Surg. 2017;104(9):1131–40. Epub 2017/06/21. PubMed PMID: 28632926. https://doi.org/10.1002/bjs.10577.

11. Li B, Yang Y, Sun Y, Hua X, Zhang X, Guo X, et al. Minimally invasive esophagectomy for esophageal squamous cell carcinoma-Shanghai Chest Hospital experience. J Thorac Dis. 2018;10(6):3800–7. https://doi.org/10.21037/jtd.2018.06.75. Epub 2018/08/03. PubMed PMID: 30069380; PMCID: PMC6051852.

12. Moon DH, Lee JM, Jeon JH, Yang HC, Kim MS. Clinical outcomes of video-assisted thoracoscopic surgery esophagectomy for esophageal cancer: a propensity score-matched analysis. J Thorac Dis. 2017;9(9):3005–12. https://doi.org/10.21037/jtd.2017.08.71. Epub 2017/12/10. PubMed PMID: 29221273; PMCID: PMC5708494.

13. Zhang X, Yang Y, Ye B, Sun Y, Guo X, Hua R, Mao T, Fang W, Li Z. Minimally invasive esophagectomy is a safe surgical treatment for locally advanced pathologic T3 esophageal squamous cell carcinoma. J Thorac Dis. 2017;9(9):2982–91. https://doi.org/10.21037/jtd.2017.07.101. Epub 2017/12/10. PubMed PMID: 29221271; PMCID: PMC5708425.

14. Tang H, Zheng H, Tan L, Shen Y, Wang H, Lin M, Wang Q. Neoadjuvant chemoradiotherapy followed by minimally invasive esophagectomy: is it a superior approach for locally advanced resectable esophageal squamous cell carcinoma? J Thorac Dis. 2018;10(2):963–72. https://doi.org/10.21037/jtd.2017.12.108. Epub 2018/04/03. PubMed PMID: 29607169; PMCID: PMC5864583.

15. Verhage RJ, Hazebroek EJ, Boone J, Van Hillegersberg R. Minimally invasive surgery compared to open procedures in esophagectomy for cancer: a systematic review of the literature. Minerva Chir. 2009;64(2):135–46. Epub 2009/04/15. PubMed PMID: 19365314.

16. Luketich JD, Pennathur A, Franchetti Y, Catalano PJ, Swanson S, Sugarbaker DJ, De Hoyos A, Maddaus MA, Nguyen NT, Benson AB, Fernando HC. Minimally invasive esophagectomy: results of a prospective phase II multicenter trial-the eastern cooperative oncology group (E2202) study. Ann Surg. 2015;261(4):702–7. https://

doi.org/10.1097/SLA.0000000000000993. Epub 2015/01/13. PubMed PMID: 25575253; PMCID: PMC5074683.

17. Ahmadi N, Crnic A, Seely AJ, Sundaresan SR, Villeneuve PJ, Maziak DE, Shamji FM, Gilbert S. Impact of surgical approach on perioperative and long-term outcomes following esophagectomy for esophageal cancer. Surg Endosc. 2018;32(4):1892–900. Epub 2017/10/27. PubMed PMID: 29067584. https://doi.org/10.1007/s00464-017-5881-6.

18. Wang J, Xu MQ, Xie MR, Mei XY. Minimally invasive Ivor-Lewis esophagectomy (MIILE): a single-center experience. Indian J Surg. 2017;79(4):319–25. https://doi.org/10.1007/s12262-016-1519-5. Epub 2017/08/23. PubMed PMID: 28827906; PMCID: PMC5549044.

19. Straatman J, van der Wielen N, Cuesta MA, Daams F, Roig Garcia J, Bonavina L, et al. Minimally invasive versus open esophageal resection: three-year follow-up of the previously reported randomized controlled trial: the TIME Trial. Ann Surg. 2017;266(2):232–6. Epub 2017/02/12. PubMed PMID: 28187044. https://doi.org/10.1097/SLA.0000000000002171.

20. Yoshida N, Yamamoto H, Baba H, Miyata H, Watanabe M, Toh Y, et al. Can minimally invasive esophagectomy replace open esophagectomy for esophageal cancer? Latest analysis of 24,233 esophagectomies from the Japanese national clinical database. Ann Surg. 2019. Epub 2019/02/06. PubMed PMID: 30720501.; https://doi.org/10.1097/sla.0000000000003222.

21. van Workum F, Stenstra M, Berkelmans GHK, Slaman AE, van Berge Henegouwen MI, Gisbertz SS, et al. Learning curve and associated morbidity of minimally invasive esophagectomy: a retrospective multicenter study. Ann Surg. 2019;269(1):88–94. Epub 2017/09/01. PubMed PMID: 28857809. https://doi.org/10.1097/SLA.0000000000002469.

22. Schmidt HM, Gisbertz SS, Moons J, Rouvelas I, Kauppi J, Brown A, et al. Defining benchmarks for transthoracic esophagectomy: a multicenter analysis of total minimally invasive esophagectomy in low risk patients. Ann Surg. 2017;266(5):814–21. Epub 2017/08/11. PubMed PMID: 28796646. https://doi.org/10.1097/SLA.0000000000002445.

23. Brierley RC, Gaunt D, Metcalfe C, Blazeby JM, Blencowe NS, Jepson M, et al. Laparoscopically assisted versus open oesophagectomy for patients with oesophageal cancer-the randomised oesophagectomy: minimally invasive or open (ROMIO) study: protocol for a randomised controlled trial (RCT). BMJ Open. 2019;9(11):e030907. Epub 2019/11/22. PubMed PMID: 31748296. https://doi.org/10.1136/bmjopen-2019-030907.

24. van Workum F, Slaman AE, van Berge Henegouwen MI, Gisbertz SS, Kouwenhoven EA, van Det MJ, et al. Propensity score-matched analysis comparing minimally invasive Ivor Lewis versus minimally invasive Mckeown esophagectomy. Ann Surg. 2018. https://doi.org/10.1097/SLA.0000000000002982. Epub 2018/08/14. PubMed PMID: 30102633.

25. Brown AM, Pucci MJ, Berger AC, Tatarian T, Evans NR 3rd, Rosato EL, Palazzo F. A standardized comparison of peri-operative complications after minimally invasive esophagectomy: Ivor Lewis versus McKeown. Surg Endosc. 2018;32(1):204–11. Epub 2017/06/24. PubMed PMID: 28643075. https://doi.org/10.1007/s00464-017-5660-4.

26. Luketich JD, Pennathur A, Awais O, Levy RM, Keeley S, Shende M, Christie NA, Weksler B, Landreneau RJ, Abbas G, Schuchert MJ, Nason KS. Outcomes after minimally invasive esophagectomy: review of over 1000 patients. Ann Surg. 2012;256(1):95–103. https://doi.org/10.1097/SLA.0b013e3182590603. Epub 2012/06/07. PubMed PMID: 22668811; PMCID: PMC4103614.

27. Deng J, Su Q, Ren Z, Wen J, Xue Z, Zhang L, Chu X. Comparison of short-term outcomes between minimally invasive McKeown and Ivor Lewis esophagectomy for esophageal or junctional cancer: a systematic review and meta-analysis. Onco Targets Ther.

2018;11:6057–69. https://doi.org/10.2147/OTT.S169488. Epub 2018/10/03. PubMed PMID: 30275710; PMCID: PMC6157998.

28. van Workum F, Berkelmans GH, Klarenbeek BR, Nieuwenhuijzen GAP, Luyer MDP, Rosman C. McKeown or Ivor Lewis totally minimally invasive esophagectomy for cancer of the esophagus and gastroesophageal junction: systematic review and meta-analysis. J Thorac Dis. 2017;9(Suppl 8):S826–S33. https://doi.org/10.21037/jtd.2017.03.173. Epub 2017/08/18. PubMed PMID: 28815080; PMCID: PMC5538973.

29. van der Werf LR, Dikken JL, van Berge Henegouwen MI, Lemmens V, Nieuwenhuijzen GAP, Wijnhoven BPL, Dutch Upper GICAg. A population-based study on lymph node retrieval in patients with esophageal cancer: results from the Dutch upper gastrointestinal cancer audit. Ann Surg Oncol. 2018;25(5):1211–20. https://doi.org/10.1245/s10434-018-6396-7. Epub 2018/03/11. PubMed PMID: 29524046; PMCID: PMC5891559.

30. Blackmon SH, Correa AM, Wynn B, Hofstetter WL, Martin LW, Mehran RJ, Rice DC, Swisher SG, Walsh GL, Roth JA, Vaporciyan AA. Propensity-matched analysis of three techniques for intrathoracic esophagogastric anastomosis. Ann Thorac Surg. 2007;83(5):1805–13. discussion 13. Epub 2007/04/28. PubMed PMID: 17462404. https://doi.org/10.1016/j.athoracsur.2007.01.046.

31. Price TN, Nichols FC, Harmsen WS, Allen MS, Cassivi SD, Wigle DA, Shen KR, Deschamps C. A comprehensive review of anastomotic technique in 432 esophagectomies. Ann Thorac Surg. 2013;95(4):1154–60. https://doi.org/10.1016/j.athoracsur.2012.11.045. discussion 60-1. Epub 2013/02/12. PubMed PMID: 23395626.

32. Ercan S, Rice TW, Murthy SC, Rybicki LA, Blackstone EH. Does esophagogastric anastomotic technique influence the outcome of patients with esophageal cancer? J Thorac Cardiovasc Surg. 2005;129(3):623–31. Epub 2005/03/05. PubMed PMID: 15746747. https://doi.org/10.1016/j.jtcvs.2004.08.024.

33. Liu YJ, Fan J, He HH, Zhu SS, Chen QL, Cao RH. Anastomotic leakage after intrathoracic versus cervical oesophagogastric anastomosis for oesophageal carcinoma in Chinese population: a retrospective cohort study. BMJ Open. 2018;8(9):e021025. https://doi.org/10.1136/bmjopen-2017-021025. Epub 2018/09/06. PubMed PMID: 30181184; PMCID: PMC6129039.

34. van der Sluis PC, Ruurda JP, van der Horst S, Goense L, van Hillegersberg R. Learning curve for robot-assisted mini-mally invasive thoracoscopic esophagectomy: results from 312 cases. Ann Thorac Surg. 2018;106(1):264–71. Epub 2018/02/20. PubMed PMID: 29454718. https://doi.org/10.1016/j.athoracsur.2018.01.038.

35. Park SY, Kim DJ, Kang DR, Haam SJ. Learning curve for robotic esophagectomy and dissection of bilateral recurrent laryngeal nerve nodes for esophageal cancer. Dis Esophagus. 2017;30(12):1–9. Epub 2017/09/09. PubMed PMID: 28881887. https://doi.org/10.1093/dote/dox094.

36. van der Sluis PC, van der Horst S, May AM, Schippers C, Brosens LAA, Joore HCA, Kroese CC, Haj Mohammad N, Mook S, Vleggaar FP, Borel Rinkes IHM, Ruurda JP, van Hillegersberg R. Robot-assisted minimally invasive thoracolaparoscopic esophagectomy versus open transthoracic esophagectomy for resectable esophageal cancer: a randomized controlled trial. Ann Surg. 2019;269(4):621–30. Epub 2018/10/12. PubMed PMID: 30308612. https://doi.org/10.1097/SLA.0000000000003031.

37. He H, Wu Q, Wang Z, Zhang Y, Chen N, Fu J, Zhang G. Short-term outcomes of robot-assisted minimally invasive esophagectomy for esophageal cancer: a propensity score matched analysis. J Cardiothorac Surg. 2018;13(1):52. https://doi.org/10.1186/s13019-018-0727-4. Epub 2018/05/25. PubMed PMID: 29792203; PMCID: PMC5967100.

38. Deng HY, Huang WX, Li G, Li SX, Luo J, Alai G, Wang Y, Liu LX, Lin YD. Comparison of short-term outcomes between robot-assisted minimally invasive esophagectomy and video-assisted minimally invasive esophagectomy in treating middle thoracic esophageal cancer. Dis Esophagus. 2018;31(8). https://doi.org/10.1093/dote/doy012. Epub 2018/03/15. PubMed PMID: 29538633.

39. Meredith K, Huston J, Andacoglu O, Shridhar R. Safety and feasibility of robotic-assisted Ivor-Lewis esophagectomy. Dis Esophagus. 2018;31(7). https://doi.org/10.1093/dote/doy005. Epub 2018/05/03. PubMed PMID: 29718160.

40. Harbison GJ, Vossler JD, Yim NH, Murayama KM. Outcomes of robotic versus non-robotic minimally-invasive esophagectomy for esophageal cancer: an American College of Surgeons NSQIP database analysis. Am J Surg. 2019;218(6):1223–8. Epub 2019/09/11. PubMed PMID: 31500797. https://doi.org/10.1016/j.amjsurg.2019.08.007.

Minimally Invasive Ivor Lewis Esophagectomy

Christopher S. Digesu and Michael Kent

There are many approaches to esophagectomy for esophageal cancer, with each offering unique advantages and disadvantages depending on cancer location, patient factors, and surgeon experience and preference. Our institution has favored the minimally invasive approach to an Ivor Lewis esophagectomy beginning with a laparoscopic intra-abdominal mobilization followed by a video-assisted thoracoscopic surgery (VATS) approach for the intrathoracic mobilization and anastomosis. This technique is particularly suited for mid to lower esophageal cancers, and while traditional teaching has been that intra-thoracic anastomoses that leak can have catastrophic complications, modern adjunctive strategies can mitigate the consequences when anastomotic leaks do occur (albeit rare) [1]. In addition, the minimally invasive technique is associated with reduced morbidity and equivalent long-term survival compared to open esophagectomy [2]. In this chapter, we discuss in detail the technical aspects of a minimally invasive Ivor Lewis esophagectomy (Video 2.1).

Patients are initially evaluated with a thorough history and physical examination. An important emphasis is placed on the nutritional and functional status of the patient as this is crucial for undergoing an esophagectomy. We do not, however, routinely place enteral access preoperatively unless patients are severely malnourished and unable to tolerate oral intake. If necessary, we prefer to place a laparoscopic jejunostomy feeding tube. Endoscopic ultrasound is routinely performed for clinical staging purposes according to

the 8th edition of the American Joint Committee on Cancer (AJCC), and a PET/CT scan is obtained to assess for metastatic disease [3]. In addition, basic laboratory values are obtained. We typically offer patients with a T1b tumor an esophagectomy, whereas patients with T2/3 or N1–2 are recommended to undergo neoadjuvant chemotherapy (carboplatin and paclitaxel) and radiation according to the CROSS trial [4]. Patients are subsequently assessed for metastatic disease via PET/CT and, if no evidence of metastatic disease, scheduled for surgery approximately 6 weeks following completion of chemoradiation.

Special Equipment

- VersaStep™ port (Medtronic, Minneapolis, MN)
- Harmonic scalpel (Ethicon, Johnson & Johnson, New Brunswick, NJ)
- Endo-GIA stapler (Medtronic, Minneapolis, MN)
- Endostitch (Medtronic, Minneapolis, MN)
- EEA stapler (Medtronic, Minneapolis, MN)

Positioning

- Preoperatively, anesthesia teams place an arterial line for close hemodynamic monitoring and a thoracic epidural for pain control.
- Antibiotics and subcutaneous heparin are administered.
- Patients are then brought to the operating room and placed in the supine position with a footboard in place and with the arms out and secured (Fig. 2.1).
- General anesthesia is induced, and patients are intubated with a left-sided double-lumen endotracheal tube.
- Bronchoscopy is performed to confirm the positioning of the endotracheal tube. The tube is taped to the patient's face on the left side of the mouth to facilitate ease of endoscopy during the case.

Electronic supplementary material The online version of this chapter (https://doi.org/10.1007/978-3-030-55669-3_2) contains supplementary material, which is available to authorized users.

C. S. Digesu
Department of Surgery, Beth Israel Deaconess Medical Center, Harvard Medical School, Boston, MA, USA

M. Kent (✉)
Department of Surgery, Division of Thoracic Surgery and Interventional Pulmonology, Beth Israel Deaconess Medical Center, Harvard Medical School, Boston, MA, USA
e-mail: mkent@bidmc.harvard.edu

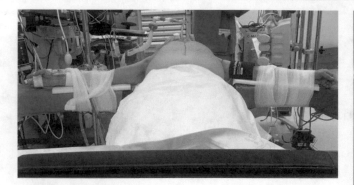

Fig. 2.1 Patients are placed in the supine position with the arms out and secured. General endotracheal anesthesia is carried out with a left-sided double-lumen endotracheal tube

- A Foley catheter is placed for urine output monitoring. The abdomen is then prepped with a chlorhexidine-based prep.
- Endoscopy is performed to confirm the location of the tumor, assess neoadjuvant response, and ensure no new abnormalities. TIP: Ensure the stomach is adequately desufflated when finished.
- Sterile drapes are placed, and the operation carried out.
- After completion of the abdominal portion of the operation, the patient is turned on the left lateral decubitus position.

Abdominal Port Placement

- First, begin with a left upper quadrant 12 mm cutdown approximately one hand's breath below the level of the costal margin. Once the peritoneum is incised, a blunt 12 mm port is placed, and the abdomen is insufflated to 12–15 mmHg.
- A left lateral 5 mm assistant port is placed, followed by a 5 mm port in the epigastrium through which a Nathanson liver retractor is placed with the post off to the patient's right side.
- A right upper quadrant 12 mm VersaStep™ port and a right lateral 5 mm subcostal port are then placed (Fig. 2.2). Tip: Use VersaStep™ to avoid having to close fascia at the end.

Mobilization of the Stomach

- Inspect the abdomen for any signs of metastatic disease using a 10 mm 30-degree laparoscope.
- The surgeon stands on the patient's right side holding an atraumatic grasper in the left hand and a laparoscopic Harmonic scalpel in the right hand. Tip: Hold the flat white blade down or toward important tissues to avoid inadvertent thermal injury.

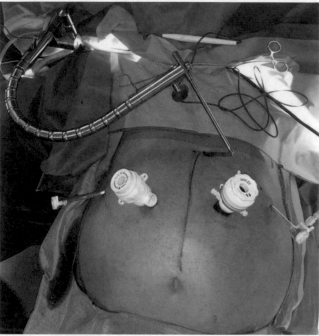

Fig. 2.2 Ports are placed as follows: 12 mm LUQ cutdown port, 5 mm LUQ subcostal port, 5 mm epigastric port to place liver retractor, 12 mm Versastep™ RUQ port, and a 5 mm right subcostal port

- The assistant stands on the patient's left side holding the camera and another atraumatic grasper to aid in retraction.
- The dissection first begins by incising the *pars flaccida* and continuing through the gastrohepatic ligament with the Harmonic scalpel heading superiorly to identify the right crus of the diaphragm. Tip: Place a 4 × 4 gauze in the abdomen to clear blood quickly and to aid in retraction.
- The assistant retracts the stomach inferiorly and to the patient's left while the surgeon uses their left-hand grasper to retract the right crus laterally dissecting into the mediastinum, being careful to avoid injury to the pleura, aorta, or pericardium.
- Dissection is carried anteriorly, incising the phrenoesophageal ligament in order to identify the left crus of the diaphragm. The esophagus is freed circumferentially.
- Next, divide the short gastric arteries. When selecting a place to begin division, it is crucial not to divide the right gastroepiploic artery. The short gastric arteries are divided at the level of the serosa of the stomach (Fig. 2.3). This makes manipulation of the stomach later in the case easier.
- Place a Penrose drain around the gastroesophageal (GE) junction.
- The stomach is elevated (retracted anteriorly), and the posterior attachments to the retroperitoneum are divided up to the level of the fundus of the stomach.

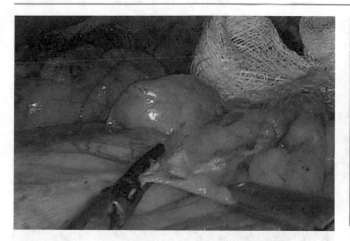

Fig. 2.3 Division of the short gastric arteries. Surgeon retracting with left hand and using Harmonic scalpel to divide directly adjacent to the serosa of the stomach

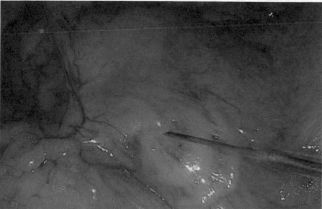

Fig. 2.5 Injection of botulinum toxin into the pylorus using a rigid injection needle

Creation of Gastric Conduit

- First, start with firing the stapler at the incisura angularis with the stapler placed through the 12 mm right upper quadrant port.
- This is facilitated by the assistant placing the stomach on stretch by grasping the fundus and pulling it toward the diaphragm. Tip: An additional port can be placed in the right lower quadrant to assist in straightening the stomach for the conduit.
- It is important to establish your trajectory, ensuring consistent sizing of the conduit with each firing of the endo-GIA stapler.
- It is also important to pay attention to the eventual margin that will be obtained.
- The conduit should be approximately 4 cm in diameter when finished (Fig. 2.6).
- We then suture the conduit to the specimen so they both can be pulled into the mediastinum. This is performed using an Endostitch device with a 0 Ethibond suture cut to 12 cm.
- The Penrose is pushed as far as it will go into the mediastinum so that it may easily be identified during the thoracoscopic portion of the case.

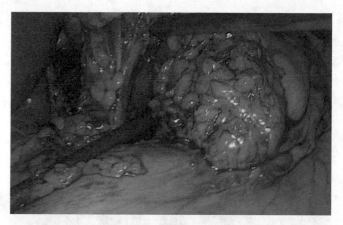

Fig. 2.4 Skeletonization of the left gastric artery which is divided with the endo-GIA stapler

- The stomach is then mobilized distally toward the duodenum to facilitate moving the stomach into the chest cavity. Tip: If the pylorus can easily reach the hiatus, then you have mobilized enough.
- Identify the left gastric artery by elevating the stomach anteriorly. The left gastric artery and vein are skeletonized and divided using a vascular load of the endo-GIA stapler (Fig. 2.4).
- Divide the right crus using the Harmonic scalpel to allow for the passage of the conduit through the hiatus.
- The last portions of the intra-abdominal mobilization include altering the pylorus to allow for adequate drainage and creating the gastric conduit. It is our practice to use botulinum toxin on the pylorus. We typically use 200 units of botulinum toxin diluted in 2 cc of normal saline injected directly into the pylorus using a rigid injection needle (Fig. 2.5).

Closing the Abdomen

- Close the left upper quadrant cutdown port site using a 0 Vicryl suture and a Carter-Thomason. The other ports are removed under direct visualization to ensure hemostasis. The skin is closed with subcuticular 4-0 Vicryl, and sterile dressings are applied.
- Prior to turning the patient, a nasogastric tube is placed.

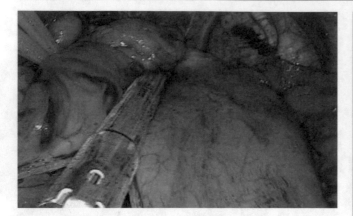

Fig. 2.6 Creation of the conduit using the endo-GIA stapler. Ensure conduit is uniform in size, ~4 cm in diameter, and an adequate margin is obtained on specimen

Right Chest: Port Placement

- Place patient on left lateral decubitus position.
- Perform a bronchoscopy at this point to ensure the endotracheal tube is in correct position.
- Gain access to chest by creating a 10 mm camera port in the anterior axillary line at approximately the level of the xiphoid.
- Place two anterior and two posterior ports to aid in dissection and retraction.

Esophageal Mobilization

- The Penrose is identified and used to elevate the esophagus out of the mediastinum.
- The inferior pulmonary ligament is divided using the Harmonic scalpel.
- Lung is retracted anteriorly using Endocinch clips (Fig. 2.7). Tip: Endocinch clips are an excellent way to maintain retraction.
- Begin with an anterior dissection of the esophagus, which is carried approximately 2 cm above the level of the azygos vein (and to ensure an adequate margin on the specimen).
- The assistant stands anterior to the patient to aid in retraction, typically with a suction instrument while also holding the camera.
- During the dissection, care is taken to avoid excessive retraction on the esophagus, to avoid thermal damage to the esophagus, and to ensure adequate hemostasis when dividing the numerous branching small vessels.
- Perform a thorough lymph node dissection with careful skeletonization of all of the subcarinal lymph nodes.
- The azygos vein is divided using the vascular load of the endo-GIA stapler (Fig. 2.8).

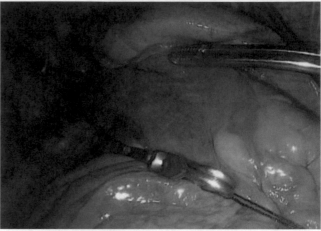

Fig. 2.7 The lung is retracted anteriorly and inferiorly to expose the esophagus. The lung is held in place using Endocinch clips. These are pulled through the anterior port and secured

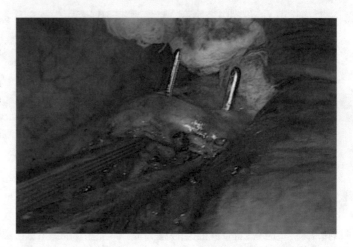

Fig. 2.8 Division of the azygous vein. This is facilitated by circumferential freeing using a right-angle forceps followed by division using the endo-GIA stapler

- The posterior plane of the esophagus is then dissected to allow for circumferential freeing of the esophagus. Lifting the Penrose helps facilitate this dissection (Fig. 2.9). Tip: When dissecting the posterior aspect, be careful to maintain a fat plane to avoid injury to the aorta or the thoracic duct.
- The specimen and conduit are pulled into view, and the Ethibond stitch placed in the abdomen is cut with laparoscopic scissors.
- The esophagus is then sharply divided at the level of the azygos vein (Fig. 2.10).
- Remove the specimen in a bag through the posterior utility port.
- The proximal margin is submitted for frozen section and confirmed to be free of malignancy prior to proceeding.

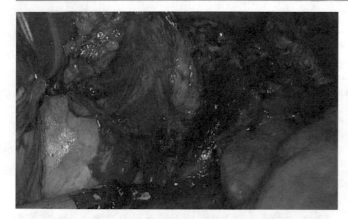

Fig. 2.9 Posterior dissection of the esophagus with the Penrose elevating the esophagus

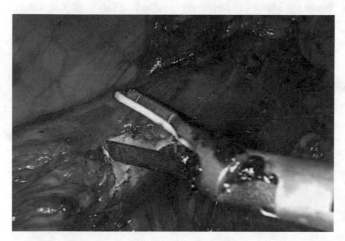

Fig. 2.10 Division of the proximal esophagus using the Harmonic scalpel

Anastomosis

- Use a 25 mm EEA stapler to create the anastomosis. Tip: May consider removing a section of the rib to ensure stapler passes into the chest easily.
- The anvil of the EEA stapler is placed in the esophageal lumen and secured with a purse-string suture.
- A gastrotomy is made with the Harmonic scalpel at the proximal end of the conduit.
- The EEA stapler is then inserted, and the spike passed through the greater curvature of the stomach.
- The EEA stapler and anvil are then mated, and the stapler is carefully fired and removed.
- The anastomotic remnants are checked to ensure they have formed an intact ring.
- The gastrotomy is then closed with a linear thoracoscopic endo-GIA stapler.
- The nasogastric tube is passed to the level of the diaphragm in the midconduit (~40 cm from the incisors).
- The chest is then irrigated with bacitracin solution.

Closing the Chest

- A 24 Fr Blake drain is placed near the anastomosis.
- The lung is visualized as the patient is placed back on two lung ventilation.
- The incisions are then sutured in standard manner.
- Sterile dressings are applied.

Postoperative Considerations

- Patients are initially maintained *nil per os* (NPO) with the nasogastric tube to low continuous suction.
- The chest tube is generally maintained to water seal, and suction is usually not needed.
- A chest x-ray is obtained in the postanesthesia care unit (PACU) to confirm positioning of all tubes, lines, and drains.
- It is our practice to maintain the patient euvolemic and avoid vasopressors in an effort to prevent conduit ischemia.
- Mobilize patients early, and they work with the physical therapy team starting on postoperative day (POD) 1.
- If they have enteral access, feeds are also initiated on postoperative day 1.
- Send a pleural fluid amylase from the pleural drain to establish a baseline.
- The nasogastric tube is removed on POD 4.
- The epidural is removed on POD 5.
- On POD 6, the patient undergoes a barium swallow. If there is no evidence of leak, we advance patients to a soft diet.
- On POD 7, if the patient is tolerating a soft diet with no concerning chest tube output and normal repeat pleural fluid amylase, we remove the chest tube.
- Depending on patient clinical and functional status, they are typically discharged on POD 7.
- Patients return to clinic 14 days following discharge with a PA and lateral chest x-ray.
- Incisions are checked for signs of infection or dehiscence, and the patient's weight and nutritional status are investigated.
- If patients had enteral access placed at the time of surgery, this is typically removed 1 month after discharge if the patient is tolerating oral intake and gain weight.

Long-Term Follow-Up

- Schedule a CT of the chest, abdomen, and pelvis at 6 months from the time of surgery for surveillance. These are continued for 2 years and then annually until 5 years.

References

1. Luketich JD, Pennathur A, Awais O, Levy RM, Keeley S, Shende M, Christie NA, Weksler B, Landreneau RJ, Abbas G, Schuchert MJ, Nason KS. Outcomes after minimally invasive esophagectomy: review of over 1000 patients. Ann Surg. 2012;256(1):95–103. https://doi.org/10.1097/SLA.0b013e3182590603. Epub 2012/06/07. PubMed PMID: 22668811; PMCID: PMC4103614.
2. Mariette C, Markar SR, Dabakuyo-Yonli TS, Meunier B, Pezet D, Collet D, D'Journo XB, Brigand C, Perniceni T, Carrere N, Mabrut JY, Msika S, Peschaud F, Prudhomme M, Bonnetain F, Piessen G, Federation de Recherche en C, French Eso-Gastric Tumors Working G. Hybrid minimally invasive esophagectomy for esophageal cancer. N Engl J Med. 2019;380(2):152–62. Epub 2019/01/10. PubMed PMID: 30625052. https://doi.org/10.1056/NEJMoa1805101.
3. Rice TW, Patil DT, Blackstone EH. 8th edition AJCC/UICC Staging of cancers of the esophagus and esophagogastric junction: application to clinical practice. Ann Cardiothorac Surg. 2017;6(2):119–30. https://doi.org/10.21037/acs.2017.03.14. Epub 2017/04/28. PubMed PMID: 28447000; PMCID: PMC5387145.
4. van Hagen P, Hulshof MC, van Lanschot JJ, Steyerberg EW, van Berge Henegouwen MI, Wijnhoven BP, Richel DJ, Nieuwenhuijzen GA, Hospers GA, Bonenkamp JJ, Cuesta MA, Blaisse RJ, Busch OR, ten Kate FJ, Creemers GJ, Punt CJ, Plukker JT, Verheul HM, Spillenaar Bilgen EJ, van Dekken H, van der Sangen MJ, Rozema T, Biermann K, Beukema JC, Piet AH, van Rij CM, Reinders JG, Tilanus HW, van der Gaast A, Group C. Preoperative chemoradiotherapy for esophageal or junctional cancer. N Engl J Med. 2012;366(22):2074–84. https://doi.org/10.1056/NEJMoa1112088. Epub 2012/06/01. PubMed PMID: 22646630.

Suggested Reading

Morse CR. Minimally invasive Ivor Lewis esophagectomy: how i teach it. Ann Thorac Surg. 2018;106(5):1283–7. Epub 2018/09/18. PubMed PMID: 30222944. https://doi.org/10.1016/j.athoracsur.2018.09.001.

Stenstra M, van Workum F, van den Wildenberg FJH, Polat F, Rosman C. Evolution of the surgical technique of minimally invasive Ivor-Lewis esophagectomy: description according to the IDEAL framework. Dis Esophagus. 2019;32(3). Epub 2018/09/25. PubMed PMID: 30247660. https://doi.org/10.1093/dote/doy079.

Tapias LF, Morse CR. Minimally invasive Ivor Lewis esophagectomy: description of a learning curve. J Am Coll Surg. 2014;218(6):1130–40. Epub 2014/04/05. PubMed PMID: 24698488. https://doi.org/10.1016/j.jamcollsurg.2014.02.014.

Minimally Invasive McKeown Esophagectomy

Matthew L. Inra and Shanda H. Blackmon

When performing a three-field minimally invasive esophagectomy, it is important to note which patients are reasonable candidates for such a procedure. Patients who have long-segment Barrett's, a middle esophageal tumor, or long length of tumor within the esophagus are ideal candidates for three-field minimally invasive esophagectomy. Patients who have an extension of disease into the cervical esophagus or tumor within the cardia of the stomach may not be ideal candidates due to an inability to create an anastomosis with this particular approach. Those patients who are thought to have extensive disease within the stomach are better candidates for laparoscopic abdominal staging and evaluation of the distal gastric conduit, and determination about whether or not a gastrectomy should be performed [1]. Patients with a low esophageal tumor and no extension into the stomach are ideal candidates for a minimally invasive Ivor Lewis esophagectomy. Patients with spine abnormalities, such as kyphosis and scoliosis, may make esophageal mobilization more difficult [2]. It is important to tailor surgery to the patient rather than the reverse.

After a complete history and physical exam, a staging of the esophageal tumor and a multidisciplinary discussion should occur to determine the most appropriate treatment algorithm [3]. After indicated neoadjuvant chemoradiotherapy or chemotherapy or chemo-immunotherapy has been delivered, the patient should be seen multiple times back in the clinic to make sure they are nutritionally optimized.

Electronic supplementary material The online version of this chapter (https://doi.org/10.1007/978-3-030-55669-3_3) contains supplementary material, which is available to authorized users.

M. L. Inra
Department of Surgery, Mayo Clinic Thoracic Surgery, Mayo Clinic Rochester, Rochester, MN, USA

Department of Cardiothoracic Surgery, Divsion of Thoracic Surgery, Lenox Hill Hospital - Northwell Health, New York, NY, USA

S. H. Blackmon (✉)
Department of Surgery, Mayo Clinic Thoracic Surgery, Mayo Clinic Rochester, Rochester, MN, USA
e-mail: blackmon.shanda@mayo.edu

Making sure that the patient's prealbumin is greater than 17, has a good performance status, has adequate pulmonary function, and is generally in an anabolic state will ensure optimal circumstances for healing postoperatively. After all these factors have been evaluated and the patient is deemed a good surgical candidate, the patient is taken to the operating room, placed in the supine position, and is endotracheally intubated under general anesthesia.

Special Equipment

- Alexis O-wound protector (Applied Medical, Rancho Santa Margarita, CA)
- Exparel liposomal bupivacaine (Pacira, Parsippany, NJ)
- Endo GIA stapler (Medtronic, Minneapolis, MN)
- Nathanson retractor (Artisan, Medford, NJ)
- Tevdek Endo Stitch device (Medtronic, Minneapolis, MN)
- LigaSure (Medtronic, Minneapolis, MN)
- TA stapler (Medtronic, Minneapolis, MN)

Positioning and Anesthesia Concerns

- Discussion at the beginning of the case, setting our expectations and making sure that all members in the operating room – surgeon, assistant, anesthesiologists, nurses – know the surgical plan.
- Discussion with anesthesia about a desire to avoid intravenous vasopressors during the case.
- If there is extension of disease close to or above the carina based on preoperative staging information, place a single-lumen endotracheal tube, and perform bronchoscopy in the operating room to ensure that there is no airway involvement, making the tumor unresectable.
- A left-sided dual-lumen endotracheal tube is placed and secured into position. A repeat bronchoscopy is performed to confirm the adequate placement of the double-lumen

endobronchial tube. Once the tube is secured, the patient is rolled into the left lateral decubitus position. All pressure points are padded. A sterile ChloraPrep (Becton, Dickinson and Company, Franklin Lakes, NJ) solution is used to prep the right hemithorax. A sterile drape around that is applied.

- After completion of right chest portion of the procedure, patient is placed on supine position.

Right Chest: Port Placement

- Four thoracoscopic port incisions are made, and the ports are placed in the chest. The ports are positioned such that two are in the anterior axillary line and two are in the posterior axillary line; the posteroinferior port is used as the utility port (Fig. 3.1) (Video 3.1). An Alexis O-wound protector is utilized for tissue retraction.
- After entering the chest cavity, we allow the lung to collapse. If necessary, use carbon dioxide insufflation to bring the lung down more rapidly.
- Place a 0 silk suture at the central tendon of the diaphragm, and bring it out of the pleural space with a trans-

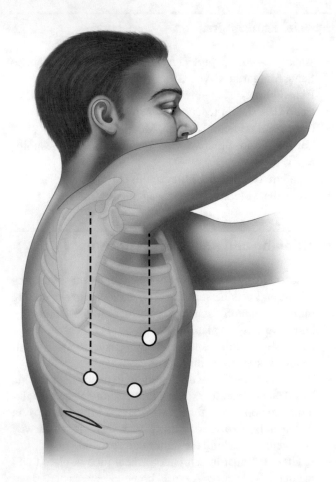

Fig. 3.1 Thoracoscopic port positioning for esophageal mobilization. The inferior posterior incision is our utility port

fascial suture passer through the chest wall; it is held in position with a hemostat, and it retracts the diaphragm in the inferior position.

- A paravertebral intercostal nerve block is employed with Exparel liposomal bupivacaine. It is injected just above the transverse process-rib junction in the intercostal space adjacent to the nerves in spaces 3 through 11. Analgesia is administered at the beginning of the case rather than at the end. The diaphragm retraction allows us to get the lower intercostal spaces.

Esophageal Mobilization and Mediastinal Lymph Node Dissection

- Inspect the base of the esophagus in the chest, which is easily done with the diaphragm retracted, and circumferentially dissect the esophagus as it exits from the hiatus. We can identify and remove stations 8 and 9 lymph nodes. Open the pleural lining along either side of the esophagus, and dissect the esophagus away from the azygos vein and the aorta, avoiding the thoracic duct.
- Evaluate for any thoracic duct injury at the time of dissection. The presence of any chyle leak or any white fluid along the posterior thoracic cavity would be worrisome for an injury. Therefore, thoracic duct ligation is not performed unless extravasation is seen in the posterior mediastinum.
- Proceed to dissect the esophagus off of the left atrium and then off of the right and left mainstem bronchi.
- Remove station 7 lymph nodes.
- Circle, staple, and divide the azygos vein with a gray load Endo GIA stapler.
- Keep a pleural tent intact superior to the azygos vein, and dissect the esophagus circumferentially proximal toward the neck.
- Divide the vagus nerves at the level of the carina, and separate them from the esophagus to prevent recurrent nerve injury from traction.
- Two Penrose drains are placed circumferentially around the esophagus to ensure complete mobilization from all attachments (Fig. 3.2a). Place one Penrose drain high along the esophagus near the thoracic inlet underneath the flap of pleural tissue that we preserved and one low toward the crura of the diaphragm to be grasped from the abdomen during the laparoscopic part of the case (Fig. 3.2b).
- After the Penrose drains are placed, a mediastinal lymph node dissection is completed. Harvest stations 4R and 10R. After all the lymph nodes are labeled as they are taken, we send them for frozen pathologic evaluation.

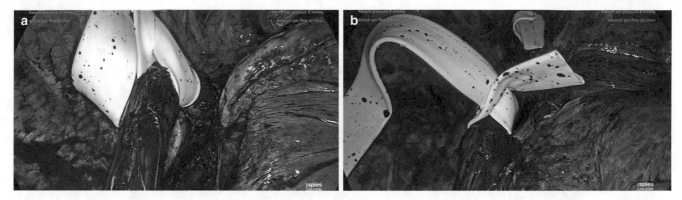

Fig. 3.2 Thoracoscopic pictures of the Penrose drains. One drain is used to circumferentially dissect the esophagus proximally toward the cervical esophagus (**a**), and the second is used to dissect distally (**b**)

Closing the Chest

- We then turn our attention toward closing the utility port in layers with 3-0 Vicryl suture (Ethicon, Johnson & Johnson, New Brunswick, NJ, USA) and 4-0 Monocryl suture (Ethicon, Johnson & Johnson, New Brunswick, NJ, USA).
- Place a chest tube exiting from the anteroinferior port, and subsequently close the other ports in layers with 3-0 Vicryl suture and 4-0 Monocryl suture. Sterile dressings are applied.
- A left-sided chest tube is also placed, usually across the right pleural space, as the two pleural cavities commonly communicate after esophageal mobilization and extensive lymph node dissection.

Abdomen: Port Placement

- The patient is undraped and repositioned supine on the operating room table. The patient's arms are tucked on both sides. Sterile ChloraPrep solution is used to prep the neck, chest, and abdominal area down to the pubis. A sterile drape around the prepped area is applied.
- Place five abdominal trocars into the abdomen. The first is a 5 mm optical trocar placed in the left subcostal region at the midclavicular line. The 10 mm port is placed at the midline above the umbilicus.
- A Nathanson retractor is placed just to the left of the xiphoid to retract the liver, and the holder is mounted to the bed (Fig. 3.3). Bovie electrocautery (Symmetry Surgical, Antioch, TN) is used to dissect through to subcutaneous tissue.
- After the abdomen is entered, the abdominal wall and peritoneal surfaces are inspected. If no metastatic disease is found after thorough laparoscopic exploration, we proceed with the remainder of the operation.
- Infusion of additional Exparel is administered at each port site for local analgesia prior to performing the rest of the procedure.

Mobilization of the Stomach

- The hepatogastric ligament is taken down with the LigaSure device.
- The hiatus of the esophagus is dissected circumferentially, taking the peritoneal lining along the right and left crural fibers as well as the phrenoesophageal membrane. This dissection leaves the raw muscular tissue of the crural fibers exposed.
- Greater curve of stomach dissection with preservation of right gastroepiploic artery. Start adjacent to the pylorus, and dissect the plane between the greater omentum and the colonic mesentery to enter the lesser sac. Start at the lateral aspect of the right gastroepiploic artery, approximately 3 cm lateral to it. Dissection is extended superiorly from there along the greater curve of the stomach, dividing the short gastric vessels to the fundus of the stomach (Fig. 3.4).
- Retract the stomach anteriorly off the pancreas, take any attachments needed to mobilize the stomach, and identify the left gastric artery and vein.
- The left gastric artery and vein pedicle are stapled and divided with a tan load Endo GIA stapler, sweeping all the lymphatic tissue up from the celiac plexus to be taken with the specimen.
- Dissect the remaining portions of the fat along the cardia of the stomach, and circumferentially dissect the esophagus, pulling the Penrose drain that had been placed in the chest down into the abdomen (Fig. 3.5).
- After the abdominal lymph node dissection is completed, mobilize the duodenum from the head of the pancreas.
- Inject 100 international units of Botox into the pylorus for improved gastric emptying postoperatively.

Creation of Gastric Conduit

- In order to create the conduit, dissect out the right gastric artery insertion point on the lesser curve of the stomach,

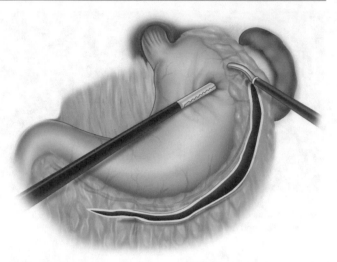

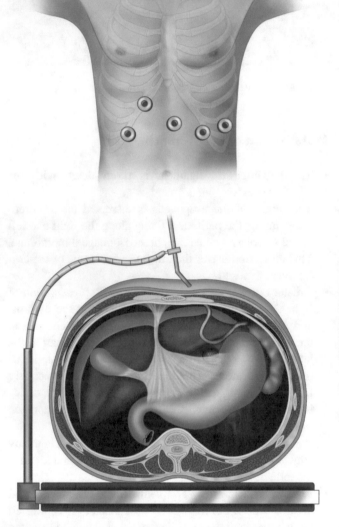

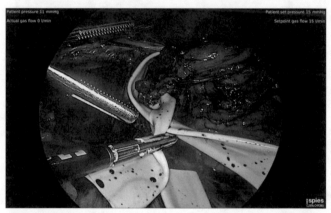

Fig. 3.4 Division of the short gastric vessels, well away from the right gastroepiploic artery. Staying away from this artery allows you to preserve the major blood supply to the conduit and create an omental flap to lay in the mediastinum and buttress your anastomosis

Fig. 3.5 Laparoscopic picture of the distal Penrose drain that is brought through the hiatus and into the abdomen. Bringing it into the abdomen ensures the esophagus and stomach are completely free prior to fashioning the conduit

Fig. 3.3 Schematic of port placement for laparoscopic dissection. If a laparoscopic liver retractor is used, generally, the superior-most port is a working port, and the most lateral port on the patient's right side is used for liver retraction (**a**). We use the Nathanson retractor that is placed in the subxiphoid position (**b**)

and just proximal to that, dissect all of the fat away from the left gastric artery branch points.

- By doing this dissection on the lesser curve of the stomach, it creates an area that is a landing zone for the purple load Endo GIA 45 mm stapler, used to initiate conduit creation. Use two of these 45 mm loads, aiming up from the lesser curve to the fundus to make a conduit that is 3.5 cm wide (Fig. 3.6).

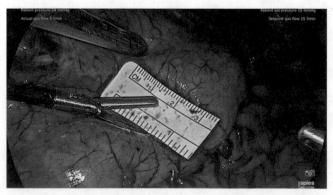

Fig. 3.6 Laparoscopic picture showing that the width of the conduit is measured using a 3.5 cm piece of measuring tape with the stapler in place at the top of the screen

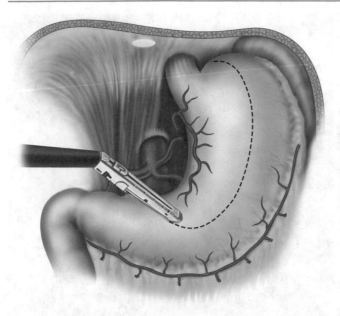

Fig. 3.7 Creation of the gastric conduit

- The beginning of the staple line is approximately at the crow's foot of the left anterior vagus nerve. Continue to create the conduit with a combination of 45 mm and 60 mm purple Endo GIA staplers, stretching and straightening the conduit as staple is applied to it to elongate and lengthen it (Fig. 3.7). Preserve several branches of the right gastric artery to optimize the conduit blood supply.
- Completely transect the specimen side of the stomach from the conduit side of the stomach.
- Reattach conduit by placing two interrupted sutures from the specimen to the tip of the conduit that is to be removed. This is done with a 2-0 Tevdek Endo Stitch device. The stomach conduit is inspected for transposition through the posterior mediastinal route and exit from the cervical incision.
- The anterior aspect of the conduit is marked with a marking pen to ensure proper orientation once it is in the neck.
- The conduit is placed into a bag before tunneling to prevent tearing of the right gastroepiploic artery as it is brought out through the neck.

Left Neck

- Create a left anterior oblique incision on the left neck along the anterior border of the sternocleidomastoid muscle with a 15-blade scalpel. Bovie electrocautery is used to dissect the subcutaneous tissue.
- The platysma muscle is divided in an oblique fashion. The tissue adjacent to the anterior border of the sternocleidomastoid is dissected with Bovie electrocautery, and then

the electrocautery is used to divide the omohyoid muscle.
- Place a thin malleable brain retractor to retract gently the esophagus and trachea medially. Using a finger and blunt Kittner dissector, develop a clear plane in the posterior space between the spine and the esophagus.
- Place a video mediastinoscope adjacent to this tissue area to facilitate the dissection of the esophagus off of the trachea while observing the recurrent laryngeal nerve and preserving it. After completing the dissection, advance the video mediastinoscope further into the mediastinum toward the right pleural space to identify the Penrose drain that had tucked previously under the pleural tent in the chest.
- Use the LigaSure to grasp the Penrose drain. Grasp the Penrose drain, and then deliver it out of the left neck, facilitating the circumferential dissection of the cervical esophagus. Keep dissection directly on the esophagus to avoid left recurrent laryngeal nerve injury or traction.
- Once this is completed, use a finger to hook around the esophagus, making sure that there is no tension or traction on the left recurrent laryngeal nerve.
- Deliver the esophagus from the neck, and complete the delivery of the specimen out of the left neck.
- The conduit is delivered into the neck in perfect orientation with the marking from the pen at 3 cm on the greater curve side of the stomach on the anterior aspect.

Anastomosis

- Perform a stapled side-to-side functional end-to-end modified Collard anastomosis of the tip of the gastric conduit to the terminal end of the esophagus with a 60 mm purple load Endo GIA stapler (Fig. 3.8a).
- Pass the nasogastric tube into the distal stomach.
- Divide the stomach and the esophageal specimen away from the stapled side-to-side anastomosis using a green load 60 mm TA stapler. The specimen is sent to frozen pathology where the proximal and distal margins are examined to ensure they are negative for tumor (Fig. 3.8b).
- Tuck the anastomosis back into the area behind the airway, ensuring the nasogastric tube is straight and not coiled within the mouth.
- Place a JP drain deep into the neck, exiting from a separate stab incision lateral to the wound.

Closure on Neck Incision

- Close the neck in layers with 3-0 Vicryl and 4-0 Monocryl interrupted suture. Interrupted sutures are important for this step because if there is a wound infection or leak, a

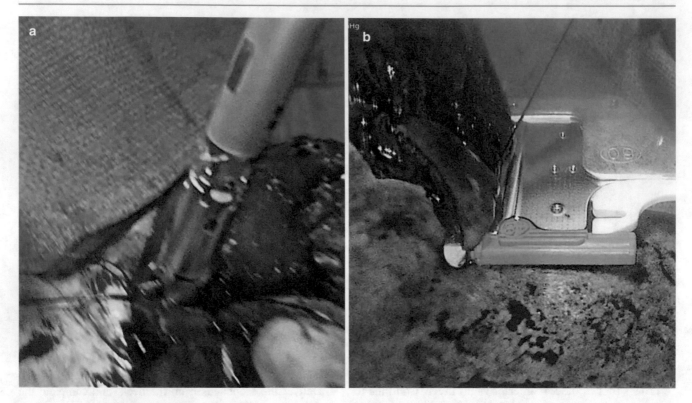

Fig. 3.8 Modified Collard esophagogastric anastomosis. Stapling of tip of gastric conduit to the terminal end of the esophagus (**a**). Closing the opening with TA stapler (**b**)

few sutures can be removed without completely opening the entire wound.

Laparoscopic Feeding Jejunostomy Tube Placement

- Place a laparoscopic feeding jejunostomy tube approximately 20 cm distal to the ligament of Treitz, bringing it up to the left anterior abdominal wall.
- Create a hand-sewn purse-string on the jejunum that is brought out onto the abdominal wall with a transfascial suture passer; it is used to pexy the jejunum to the anterior abdominal wall.
- Tack the jejunum into position with additional T-fasteners. Inspect the intraperitoneal surface to make sure that there is no tension on the jejunum.

Closure of Abdomen

- Check that the duodenum is in proper position, that there is no bleeding in the splenic bed, and that all of the sponges and instruments have been removed.
- Close the 10 mm abdominal port with a transfascial suture passer utilizing 0 Vicryl suture.

- All sponge and instrument counts are confirmed to be correct upon completion of the surgery and before closure of the abdomen.
- A left-sided Blake drain is placed into the chest to drain the fluid, if it was not placed transpleurally already, and it is sutured in place with 0 silk suture.

Postoperative Considerations

- Patients are kept NPO for 1 month after surgery.
- Tube feeds begin once bowel function returns.
- Fluids are administered as needed, and a low maintenance rate is maintained for resuscitation.
- Heparin or low-molecular-weight heparin is used for DVT prophylaxis.
- Early ambulation and use of an incentive spirometer are emphasized.
- A postesophagectomy enhanced recovery pathway is utilized. Typically, the nasogastric tube is removed on postoperative day 7.
- Twenty-four hours of observation allow the team to ensure that no leak is present after the nasogastric tube is removed and there is not conduit distension, and the pleural drains are then removed.

- Patients are typically discharged on postoperative day 8. Patients are encouraged to return when they are exactly 1 month out from surgery for a contrast esophagram and to begin an oral diet if no leak is identified.

References

1. Bonavina L, Incarbone R, Lattuada E, Segalin A, Cesana B, Peracchia A. Preoperative laparoscopy in management of patients with carcinoma of the esophagus and of the esophagogastric junction. J Surg Oncol. 1997;65(3):171–4. Epub 1997/07/01. PubMed PMID: 9236925. https://doi.org/10.1002/(sici)1096-9098(199707)65:3<171::aid-jso5>3.0.co;2-3.
2. Okamura A, Watanabe M, Mine S, Nishida K, Imamura Y, Kurogochi T, Kitagawa Y, Sano T. Factors influencing difficulty of the thoracic procedure in minimally invasive esophagectomy. Surg Endosc. 2016;30(10):4279–85. Epub 2016/01/09. PubMed PMID: 26743111. https://doi.org/10.1007/s00464-015-4743-3.
3. Basta YL, Bolle S, Fockens P, Tytgat K. The value of multidisciplinary team meetings for patients with gastrointestinal malignancies: a systematic review. Ann Surg Oncol. 2017;24(9):2669–78. https://doi.org/10.1245/s10434-017-5833-3. Epub 2017/03/25. PubMed PMID: 28337661; PMCID: PMC5539280.

Suggested Reading

Perry Y, Fernando HC. Three-field minimally invasive esophagectomy: current results and technique. J Thorac Cardiovasc Surg. 2012;144(3):S63–6. Epub 2012/06/30. PubMed PMID: 22743173. https://doi.org/10.1016/j.jtcvs.2012.06.002.

Robot-Assisted Ivor Lewis Esophagectomy

David C. Rice

Esophageal carcinoma is the eighth most common cancer worldwide and the sixth most common cause of cancer-related death [1]. Although squamous cell carcinoma (ESCC) represents the most common histology, in the United States and many other Western countries, the incidence rate of adenocarcinoma (EAC) now exceeds that of ESCC, and this is expected to only increase [2]. Most EACs affect the lower third of the esophagus and gastroesophageal junction, and since the location of these tumors generally does not require removal of the entire esophagus, partial esophagectomy with intrathoracic anastomosis is increasingly favored among thoracic surgeons. Furthermore, the majority of surgically resectable patients present with locoregionally advanced stage requiring induction chemo- or chemoradiation therapy up front, which may lessen the reliability of the stomach conduit for anastomosis in the neck. Therefore, over the last decade, there has been a shift in the approach to esophagectomy away from transhiatal and three-hole (McKeown) techniques toward a transthoracic (Ivor Lewis) approach [3]. Furthermore, this trend has been observed for both open esophagectomy and minimally invasive esophagectomy (MIE). Because performance of MIE with intrathoracic anastomosis is technically complex, particularly with respect to the performance of the anastomosis, the advent of robotics has delivered greater dexterity with a minimally invasive approach and may overcome some of the technical limitations inherent in "straight stick" laparoscopic/thoracoscopic approaches. A recent consensus statement recommended standardizing the nomenclature for esophagectomy according to procedure and approach; therefore, robotic-assisted Ivor Lewis esophagectomy is referred to as ILER [4].

Electronic supplementary material The online version of this chapter (https://doi.org/10.1007/978-3-030-55669-3_4) contains supplementary material, which is available to authorized users.

D. C. Rice (✉)
Department of Thoracic and Cardiovascular Surgery, Division of Surgery, University of Texas MD Anderson Cancer Center, Houston, TX, USA
e-mail: drice@mdanderson.org

The majority of patients will be candidates for ILER. However, consideration should be given to the following patient-related factors:

Obesity Patients who are obese are certainly more technically challenging than nonobese patients. This is especially a factor during the identification of the lesser sac, during the dissection of the omentum away from the greater curvature of the stomach, and in the creation of the omental flap. Patient obesity obscures planes and makes exposure difficult. Adequate decompression of the stomach with a well-placed and functional nasogastric tube, utilizing a bedside assistant to aid in retraction and exposure, placement of the patient (well-secured) in steep reverse Trendelenburg position, and use of bariatric trocars may facilitate the procedure. The trade-off regarding obese patients is that visualization of the upper abdomen is often superior during minimally invasive esophagectomy compared to an open esophagectomy. Additionally, it is rare for patients to develop postoperative wound infections.

Preoperative Therapy The majority of patients will have received induction treatment, usually concurrent chemoradiation. This rarely presents a challenge, certainly if the surgery is within a month or two of the completion of therapy. Beyond 3 months, there seems to be an increased tendency for fibrotic adhesions. Despite making identification of the correct planes of dissection surgery more difficult, even salvage procedures are usually technically feasible.

Previous Gastrostomy Tube These generally are placed in the antrum of the stomach and invariably exit on the greater curvature close to the course of the right gastroepiploic artery (RGEA). Though the robot is helpful in meticulously dissecting out and closing the gastrostomy, great care must be taken to preserve the RGEA. If the artery is injured or not viable, an alternate conduit may need to be considered. In

M. P. Kim (ed.), *Atlas of Minimally Invasive and Robotic Esophagectomy*, https://doi.org/10.1007/978-3-030-55669-3_4

general, I prefer to place a feeding jejunostomy laparoscopically if there is a need for preoperative nutritional supplementation.

Tumor Size/Extent Larger tumors tend to be more difficult to dissect, particularly at the level of the hiatus; however, they are not usually a contraindication to a robotic approach. Clinical suspicion of aortic involvement should obviously contraindicate a robotic approach. However, the diaphragmatic invasion may often be successfully tackled with resection of a cuff of the diaphragm.

Previous Abdominal Operations Previous lower abdominal procedures usually have a negligible effect on the performance of ILER; however, as with open esophagectomy, previous upper abdominal surgery will complicate exposure and conduct of the procedure. The enhanced ability to visualize appropriate tissue planes and to meticulously dissect when using the robot often enables ILER to be successfully performed even after previous upper abdominal surgeries, e.g., laparotomy for a gunshot wound to the abdomen, transverse colectomy, fundoplication, etc. Although there is little downside to embarking on a minimally invasive approach, one's threshold to convert to laparotomy should be low if progress and safety are jeopardized by scarring and inability to visualize anatomy.

Patients are managed according to an enhanced recovery after surgery (ERAS) pathway. Because of the possibility of esophageal obstruction and aspiration, patients are fasting from midnight before surgery. Preoperative analgesics, including tramadol ER 300 mg and gabapentin 300 mg, are orally administered in the holding area.

Special Equipment

- Exparel® liposomal bupivacaine (Pacira Inc., Parsippany, New Jersey)
- FreeHold Trio™ (FreeHold Surgical, New Hope, Pennsylvania)
- V-Loc™ (Covidien, Dublin, Ireland)
- STRATAFIX™ (Johnson & Johnson, New Brunswick, New Jersey)
- Da Vinci Xi robot
  - Tip-up fenestrated grasper or grasping retractor (Small Graptor™)
  - Vessel sealer
  - Curved bipolar dissector
  - Fenestrated bipolar forceps
  - Monopolar curved scissors

- Mega SutureCut™ Needle Driver
- Robotic stapler – SureForm ™ 60 instrument with 2.5 mm (white), 3.5 mm (blue), and 4.3 mm (green) loads

Positioning and Anesthesia Concerns

- Patient is initially placed in a supine position and a general anesthetic is administered.
- Two large-bore intravenous lines are established. There is no routine need for central venous catheters.
- Arterial line and urinary catheter are placed because of the length of the case and potential for fluid shifts during the case.
- A double-lumen endotracheal tube for single lung ventilation during the thoracic phase of the procedure
- Combined use of inhalational and intravenous anesthetics is routinely employed along with bispectral monitoring of brain wave activity.
- A silicone nasogastric tube is placed.
- Esophagoscopy is selectively performed to confirm preoperative estimates of tumor location and extent and assess mucosal viability following preoperative radiotherapy.
- Liposomal bupivacaine is used to enhance postoperative pain management. Liposomal bupivacaine of 266 mg is diluted to a final volume of 80 cc using normal saline. At the conclusion of the abdominal phase, 40 cc is infiltrated around the abdominal port sites. The remainder is used to infiltrate the incisions during the thoracic phase.
- The arms are tucked at the side, and the patient is placed in a slight reverse Trendelenburg position (20°–25°), and a footboard is placed. Some authors also recommend rotating the table 10° to the patient's right side [5].
- The abdomen should be prepared widely on each side, especially on the left as the left-sided ports may extend laterally beyond the midaxillary line. The cranio-caudad extent of the sterile field should be from at least the level of the nipples to the pubis.
- After completion of the abdominal portion of the operation, the patient is turned in a left lateral decubitus position.

Abdominal Port Placement

- The basic principles regarding port placement are to ensure enough separation between ports (at least 8–10 cm) to avoid placing ports too caudally as this can limit the ability to dissect far into the hiatus. In general, four robotic ports will be used that include a 12 mm trocar for stapling/dissection and three 8 mm trocars for the camera

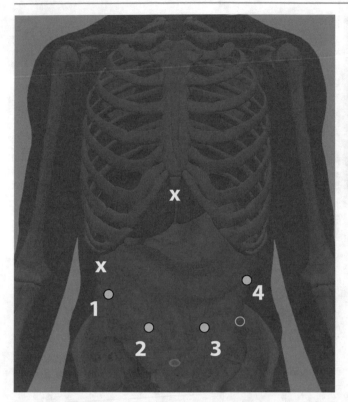

Fig. 4.1 Port placement for abdominal phase. Numbers refer to the robotic arms. Arm 1, 12 mm port; Arms 2–4, 8 mm ports. X refers to site of Nathanson (subxiphoid) or laparoscopic (right flank) liver retractors. Open circle is the assist port (optional)

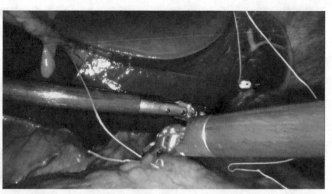

Fig. 4.2 Intracorporeal retraction of the left lobe of the liver (FreeHold Trio™) avoids additional ports for external retractors

and dissection/retraction (Fig. 4.1) (Video 4.1). I do not routinely place an assist trocar; however, in the case of bleeding or if additional retraction is needed, a 5 mm assist port is added.

- Place the ports in a gentle curve with its nadir about 2 cm cephalad to the umbilicus.
  - 12 mm port (Arm 1) in the right upper quadrant in the midclavicular line
  - 8 mm port (Arm 2) in the paramedian position about 2 cm cephalad and to the right of the umbilicus which will be used for the camera
  - 8 mm port in a left paramedian position (Arm 3)
  - 8 mm port in a left subcostal position (Arm 4)
  - 5 mm assist port (optional), usually between Arms 3 and 4.
- Retraction is provided using the tip-up grasper or the small grasping retractor (Graptor™) which is placed in either Arm 1 or Arm 4, depending on whether the camera is placed in Arm 2 or Arm 3.
  - For initial dissection, I typically place the camera in Arm 2 and retract with Arm 4.
  - When dissecting up along the greater curvature toward the left side of the hiatus, hiatus visualization is often facilitated by moving the camera to Arm 3 and placing the retractor in Arm 1, using Arms 2 and 4 to dissect.

- The nondominant and dominant instruments are placed in ports on either side of the camera port.
  - The nondominant hand instrument is usually the fenestrated bipolar grasper, robotic stapler, and occasionally the vessel sealer.
  - The dominant hand instruments are the curved bipolar dissector and the vessel sealer.

Liver Retraction

- Place a Nathanson liver retractor or laparoscopic fan retractor (or similar device) for retraction of the left lobe of the liver.
  - Although both provide adequate exposure, they require an additional port/incision and are externally supported which can sometimes interfere with the range of mobility of the robotic arms.
- Currently, I prefer totally intracorporeal retractors such as the Freehold Trio™ (FreeHold Surgical, New Hope, Pennsylvania) which provides excellent retraction and may be easily deployed through an existing 8 mm port (Fig. 4.2).

Dissection of Greater Curve and Creation of the Omental Flap

- A pedicled omental flap is harvested for later use in buttressing the anastomosis in the chest. The flap should ideally be based on one or two omental branches off the RGEA.
  - Do not use the entire omentum as this is often substantial in size and may result in compression of the lung and atelectasis (Fig. 4.3a).
- Identify the pedicled blood supply. The omentum is divided lateral to the vessels on either side, entering the lesser sac.

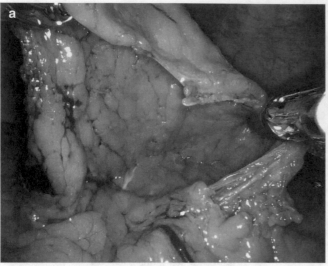
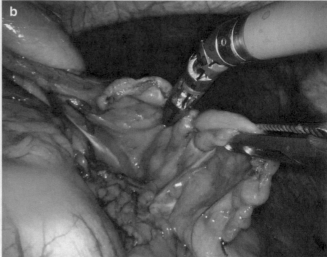

Fig. 4.3 (**a**) Dissection begins by elevating the greater omentum off the colon and creating a flap based on omental branches of the right gastroepiploic artery (RGEA). (**b**) Dissection proceeds along the greater curvature of the stomach using the vessel sealer to divide the omentum approximately 2 cm away from the course for the RGEA

- Elevate the omentum cephalad, and the attachments to the colon and mesentery are taken down using bipolar electrocautery.
  - Care should be taken to avoid dissecting the omentum too close to the course of the RGEA to avoid injury to the blood supply of the conduit (Fig. 4.3b).

Mobilization of Stomach

- After the flap has been harvested, divide the omentum heading cephalad along the greater curvature of the stomach using the vessel sealer.
- Visualize the course of the RGEA, and keep at least 2 cm off the greater curvature to avoid inadvertent injury.
  - Use of indocyanine green may be helpful in demonstrating the RGEA, especially in identifying unseen collateral vessels from the distal RGEA that may course through the greater curvature tissue and anastomose with the short gastric arteries [6].
- Retract the stomach further to the right and elevate anteriorly, and divide the short gastric vessels to the level of the left crus (Fig. 4.4a).
  - Placement of the camera in Arm 3 using Arm 1 for retraction is often helpful.
  - Additionally, downward retraction of the splenic flexure or pancreas by the bedside assistant is often helpful, particularly in obese patients.
- Elevate the stomach anteriorly, and identify the plane between the omentum and colonic mesentery.
  - Attachments of the mesentery to the posterior stomach are taken down (Fig. 4.4b).

- Divide the omental attachments at the proximal greater curvature using the vessel sealer (Fig. 4.4c).
- Identify the RGEA pedicle and trace proximally to its origin with the gastroduodenal artery.
  - Once this has been determined, divide any additional omental tissue anterior to the RGEA pedicle to the level of first portion of the duodenum (Fig. 4.4e).
- Perform a Kocher maneuver to allow reach of the conduit into the chest.

Mobilization of Stomach, Mobilization of Esophagus, and Dissection of Lesser Curve

- Incise the lesser omentum close to the liver using bipolar energy and dividing the gastrohepatic ligament until the right crus is identified (Fig. 4.5a).
  - The absence of a replaced left hepatic artery is established (see below).
- Mobilize the right crus away from the abdominal esophagus.
  - Place FreeHold liver retractor at this time.
- Divide the phrenoesophageal ligament anterior to the esophagus until the anterior left crus is reached (Fig. 4.5b).
- Divide the lesser omentum from its attachment to the stomach at the incisura angularis, laterally cephalad to the right gastric artery (RGA).
  - This is a vascular region and is best approached by careful dissection between vessels on the wall of the stomach with the curved bipolar dissector, creating a tunnel and then completing the division of the lesser curve tissue with serial applications of the vessel sealer (Fig. 4.5c).

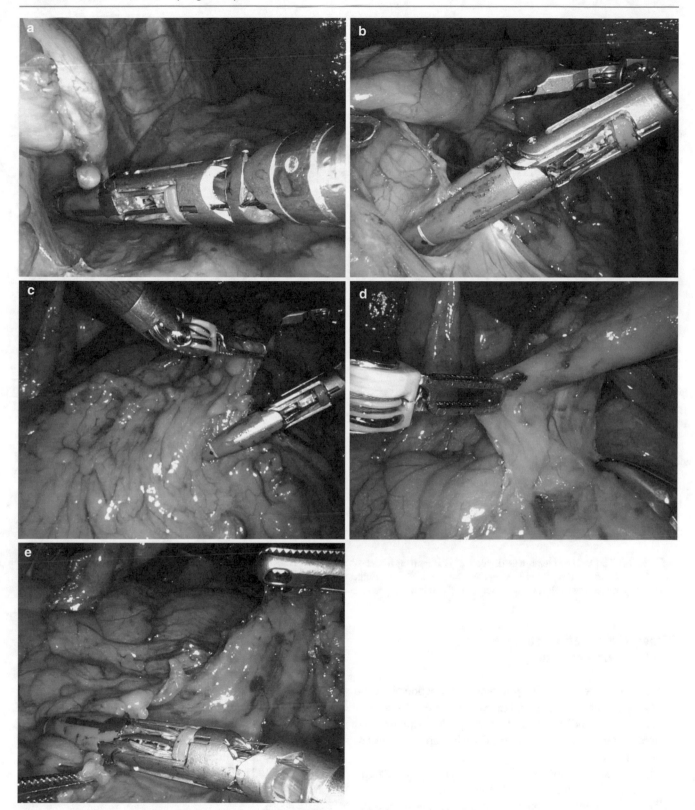

Fig. 4.4 (**a**) With the stomach being retracted leftward, dissection continues until the left crus is reached. The peritoneum is divided anteriorly to the level of the phrenoesophageal ligament. (**b**) Posterior attachments between the stomach and colon or colonic mesentery are divided. (**c**) The omentum is divided to the right of the omental flap along the course of the RGEA. (**d**) The course of the RGEA is traced proximally to its origin with the gastroduodenal artery. Bipolar electrocautery is used to avoid injury to the vessels. (**e**) Omental tissue anterior to the RGEA may be divided to the level of the first portion of the duodenum

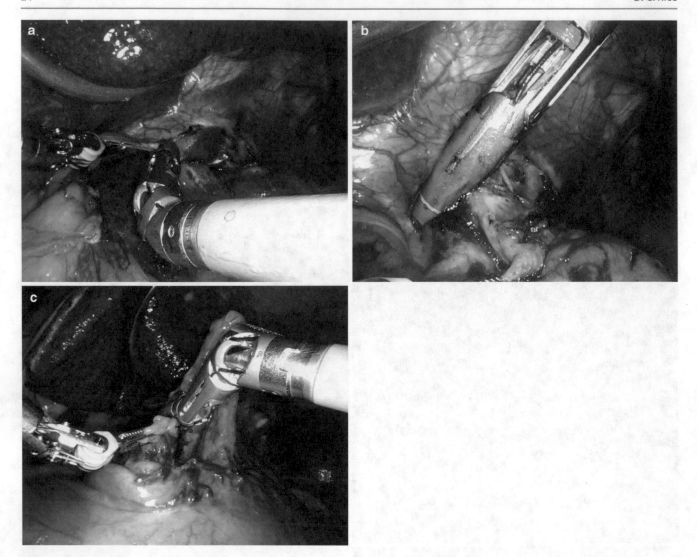

Fig. 4.5 (**a**) The lesser omentum is divided. It is important to determine the existence of a replaced left hepatic artery, which, if present, will modify division of the left gastric artery. (**b**) The phrenoesophageal ligament is divided exposing the right crus. (**c**) The lesser curve tissue is divided at the level of the incisura angularis. The right gastric artery is preserved

Dissection of Left Gastric Vessels and Lymphadenectomy

- Perform a "modified" D2 lymph node dissection using the curved bipolar dissector and the vessel sealer. It is considered a "modified' D2 dissection as the gastroepiploic and greater curvature nodes and right gastric artery nodes are not removed.
- Identify the common hepatic artery and dissect the porta hepatic nodal tissue anterior to the artery.
- Trace the common hepatic artery proximally toward the celiac trunk.
  - Care should be taken not to dissect into the pancreas as the tissue may look like a lymph node.
- Identify the coronary or left gastric vein (LGV), skeletonize, and then divide with a vessel sealer (Fig. 4.6a, b).
- Divide the tissue medial to the artery and superficial to the head of the pancreas.

- Identify the left gastric artery which is typically found just cephalad to the LGV (Fig. 4.6c).
- Dissect the lymph node station around the left gastric artery.
- Skeletonize left gastric artery to its origin with the celiac trunk and divide with a 60 mm robotic stapler with white cartridge (2.5 mm) (Fig. 4.6d).
- Dissect the fatty and lymphatic tissue on the left side of the artery, continuing the plane of dissection anterior and cephalad to the pancreas along the proximal splenic artery, eventually turning toward the left crus (Fig. 4.6e).
- Remove the celiac axis nodal tissue.
- Gently retract the common hepatic artery (CHA) inferiorly, and remove the nodal tissue cephalad to the CHA, portal vein, lateral to the celiac trunk and superficial to the inferior vena cava (Fig. 4.6f).

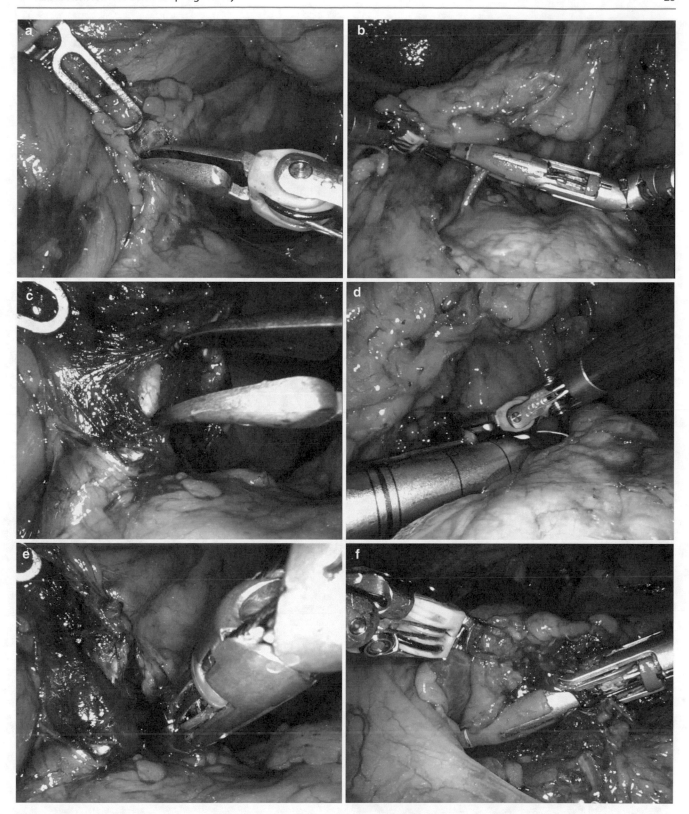

Fig. 4.6 (a) The stomach is elevated anteriorly and the left gastric (coronary) vein is dissected. (b) Division of the left gastric vein with the vessel sealer. (c) The left gastric artery is dissected free of tissue using the curved bipolar dissector. (d) The left gastric artery is divided with a robotic linear stapler with 2.5 mm (white) staple cartridge. (e) Tissue medial to the left gastric artery and along the dorsal surface of the pancreas and splenic artery is divided. (f) Nodal tissue lateral to the celiac axis, cephalad to the proper hepatic artery and portal vein, and superficial to the inferior vena cava is resected

Creation of the Gastric Conduit

- Dissect the posterior surface of the stomach and esophagus into the lower mediastinum, on the anterior surface of the descending thoracic aorta, and once the left gastric vessels have been divided, the stomach is elevated anteriorly.
- Create a narrow stomach tube, around 4–5 cm in width (which promotes improved gastric drainage).
  - Start at the incisura angularis and taking serial firings of the 60 mm robotic linear stapler using either blue (3.5 mm) or green (4.3 mm) cartridges, depending on the observed thickness of the stomach (Fig. 4.7a).
  - Stretch out the stomach as long as possible along its axis.

- This is most easily achieved by using the retraction instrument to bluntly distract the antrum inferiorly while the surgeon's right hand pulls inferiorly on the divided lesser curve tissue (Fig. 4.7b).
- Pass the stapler through the 12 mm port (Arm 1) and control it by the surgeon's left hand.
- Completely divide the stomach at the level of the cardia (Fig. 4.7c).
- Reflect the conduit to the left of the patient, exposing the posterior surface of the antrum.
- Further mobilize the posterior attachments to the level of the pylorus.
- Inject ICG (12.5 mg – half of a 10 cc vial) and assess the perfusion of the conduit.
  - Administer ICG intravenously by bolus injection and assess the quality of the perfusion of the conduit using

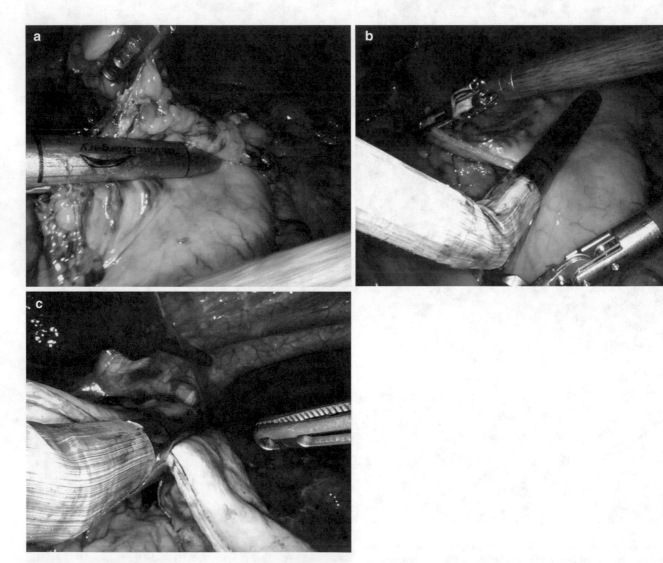

Fig. 4.7 (a) The conduit is created using a robotic linear stapler, beginning at the incisura angularis. 3.5 mm (blue) or 4.3 mm (green) staple cartridges are used. Care must be taken to ensure the nasogastric tube has been fully withdrawn first. (b) A narrow (4–5 cm) conduit is created. The stomach is elongated during stapling using rightward retraction on the lesser curve (Arm 3) and blunt caudal retraction on the conduit (Arm 4). (c) The stomach is completely divided at the cardia, lateral to the phrenoesophageal fat

near-infrared imaging by turning on the Firefly function on the Xi robot console (Fig. 4.8a).

- If there is any ischemic area, mark the area of demarcation with a silk stitch so that an anastomosis may be avoided in this area (Fig. 4.8b, c).

Pyloric Drainage Procedure

- Debate continues regarding the necessity for a pyloric drainage procedure following esophagectomy with some studies showing it to be unnecessary and others showing higher rates of aspiration, delayed gastric emptying, or anastomotic leak [7–10]. Nonetheless, pyloric injection of botulinum toxin is simple to perform and may decrease rates of delayed gastric emptying, though its efficacy remains unproven [11, 12].

- In my practice, I inject botulinum toxin in the pylorus.
  - Dilute 200 IU botulinum toxin A in total of 5 cc. Note, 1 cc of solution is needed to preload the needle channel.
  - Inject 1 cc in four quadrants around the pylorus using a flexible, retractable colonoscopy needle through one of the ports. Once the conduit has been created, access to the posterior aspect of the pylorus is straightforward (Fig. 4.9).

Hiatal Dissection

- Retract the divided proximal stomach and abdominal esophagus to allow further circumferential dissection into the mediastinum (Fig. 4.10a).
  - Maintain maximal radial margins.

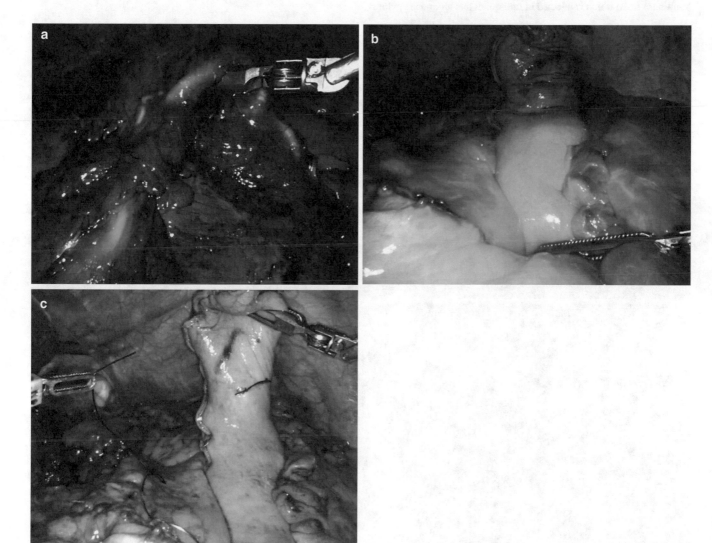

Fig. 4.8 (a) Bolus intravenous injection of 12.5 mg indocyanine green (IGC) is performed, which highlights the course of the RGEA using near-infrared imaging (Firefly). (b) A relatively ischemic area at the tip of the conduit may be often identified. (c) The region of malperfusion may be marked with a suture to ensure placement of the anastomosis at a well-vascularized portion of the conduit

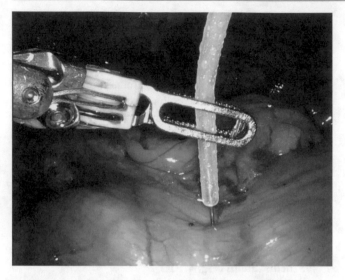

Fig. 4.9 A "chemical pyloromyotomy" is performed using 200 IU botulinum toxin which is injected in four quadrants around the pylorus

– The planes of dissection included the adventitia of the aorta inferiorly, the pleura bilaterally, and the posterior pericardium anteriorly. It is typical that one or both pleural spaces are entered. The esophagus is dissected up into the chest usually to 2–3 cm below the carina (Fig. 4.10b, c).
– Care must be taken to avoid injury to the inferior pulmonary veins which may be encountered anterolaterally on either side in continuity with the pericardium.
- Suture the tip of the conduit to the remaining divided lesser curve tissue using a 2-0 silk suture.
- Suture the omental flap secured to the lesser curve in a similar manner (Fig. 4.11).
- Ensure that the conduit lays in an orthogonal position without any twisting.

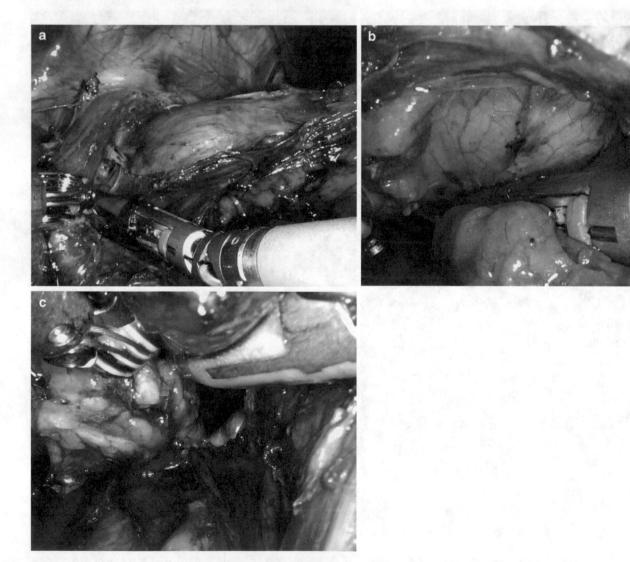

Fig. 4.10 (a) The esophagus is circumferentially dissected into the mediastinum attempting to keep wide radial margins. (b) The anterior plane of dissection is along the posterior pericardium. (c) The posterior plane of dissection is along the anterior border of the descending thoracic aorta. Laterally, the pleura is usually entered on either side to ensure maximum margins

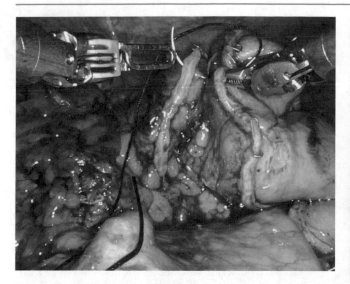

Fig. 4.11 The conduit and omental flap are sutured to the remaining divided curve tissue so that they may be easily delivered into the chest during the thoracic phase

Jejunostomy Tube

- A jejunostomy feeding tube is not typically placed unless there are concerns regarding the viability of the stomach conduit or other expectation of need for prolonged supplemental enteral nutrition [13].
- However, it is prudent to identify a limb of proximal jejunum and tack this to the anterior abdominal wall in the left upper quadrant, marking its position with titanium clips. This will enable the interventional radiologist to access to the upper jejunum percutaneously using fluoroscopy and placement of a feeding tube if it necessary, such as in the case of an anastomotic leak.
- Suture the jejunum to the abdominal wall using silk sutures to prevent torsion.
- Alternatively, a nasojejunal feeding tube may be placed at the end of the case and directed across the pylorus with an endoscope. However, this requires the patient to endure two nasogastric tubes, which is uncomfortable and, in my experience, usually unnecessary.

Patient Positioning for Thoracic Phase

- Position the patient in a left lateral decubitus position and flexed.
- Place the table in a slight reverse Trendelenburg (20°–25°) to facilitate egress of the diaphragm.
- Rotate the patient slightly prone which helps with the lung retraction away from the esophagus.
- Certain experts recommend a more pronounced prone positioning (e.g., 45° rotation anteriorly); however, this limits the ability to place the larger 12 mm trocar anteriorly where the intercostal spaces are wider [5].

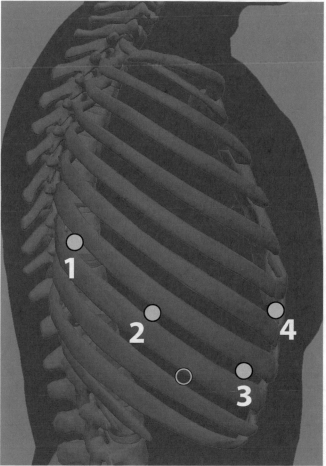

Fig. 4.12 Port placement for thoracic phase. Numbers refer to the robotic arms. Arms 1, 2, and 4 8 mm ports; Arm 3, 12 mm port. Open circle indicates site of assistant port (optional)

Thoracic Port Placement

- Four robotic ports are placed following the ribs, usually in the 8th or 9th intercostal spaces. The precise position of the ports will vary depending on body habitus (Fig. 4.12).
- Place three ports spaced pit along the 8th or 9th intercostal spaces, from posterior to anterior:
  - Arm 1: 8 mm port, anterior to paraspinal muscles (left-hand instrument)
  - Arm 2: 8 mm port, midaxillary line (camera)
  - Arm 3: 12 mm port, anterior to anterior axillary line (stapler, right-hand instrument)
  - Arm 4: 8 mm port 1 or 2 interspaces above and anterior to Arm 3 (lung and esophagus retraction)
- If an assist port is required, it may be placed between Arm 2 and Arm 3 and used as an extraction site for the chest drain.
- Insufflate the chest with warm CO_2 to a pressure of 5–10 mmHg to help displace and flatten the diaphragm inferiorly.

Division of Pleura and Azygos Vein

- Usually, the right pleura will have already been entered during the abdominal phase of the dissection.
- Continue the pleural dissection anterior to the esophagus along the pericardium posterior to the right inferior pulmonary vein using the vessel sealer (Fig. 4.13a).
- At the level of the inferior border of the right main bronchus (RMB), use bipolar electrocautery to minimize the risk or thermal injury to the airway (Fig. 4.13b).
- Dissect the pleura to the azygos vein, and then divide the pleura along the inferior edge of the azygos vein.
- Skeletonize the azygos vein as it crosses over the right main bronchus and divide with a linear robotic stapler (SureForm™ 60 instrument, white 2.5 mm load) (Fig. 4.13c).

Lymphadenectomy

- Remove periesophageal and inferior pulmonary ligament nodes en bloc with the specimen.
- Resect the subcarinal nodes and those along the distal RMB (10R) lymph nodes (Fig. 4.14a).
  - These are often quite well perfused from bronchial and esophageal arteries arising from the aorta. I have found that it is often best to dissect the nodes from posterior to anterior, creating a plane between the esophagus and the node, cauterizing and dividing the vessels as they are encountered (Fig. 4.14b).
  - The posterior and inferior aspect of the left main bronchus (LMB) will be encountered, and bipolar electrocautery should be used to minimize risk of injury.
  - Once the posterior vascular attachments of the subcarinal node have been divided, the node may be dissected

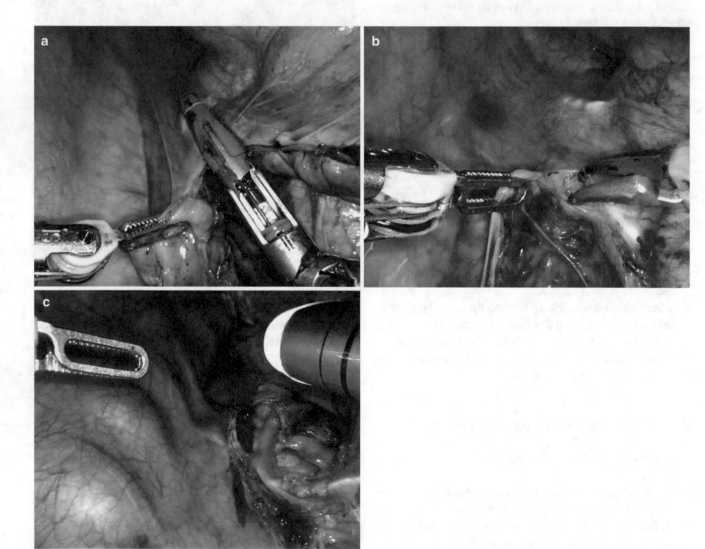

Fig. 4.13 (a) Anterior pleura is divided, excising all tissue posterior to the pericardium en bloc with esophagus. (b) At the level of the right main bronchus, dissection proceeds with bipolar electrocautery to avoid thermal injury to membranous airway. (c) The azygos vein is divided with a linear robotic stapler using either 2.0 mm (gray) or 2.5 mm (white) staple cartridges

from anterior to posterior along the inferior RMB and the pericardium, inferiorly. There is usually an arterial branch that enters the node deep to the carina, and this should be anticipated and cauterized, which is usually safe to do as the LMB has already been identified and separated from the nodal packet (Fig. 4.14c).

- The nodal specimen is removed with a specimen retrieval bag through the 12 mm port (Arm 2).

- Unless there is radiologic or endoscopic suspicion of involvement preoperatively, a paratracheal nodal dissection is not usually performed, although some surgeons perform this routinely [14].

Posterior Esophageal Dissection

- Dissect the pleura posteriorly along the vertebra following the course of the azygos vein (Fig. 4.15a, b).

- If en bloc esophagectomy is performed with removal of the thoracic duct along with the specimen, the duct is initially ligated and divided at the level of the hiatus.
  - The anterolateral aspect of the descending aorta is usually visible from the previous abdominal dissection.
  - Identify the prevertebral fascia and the segmental intercostal arteries and veins. A plane is established between anterior aspect of the vertebra and connects with the adventitial plane on the aorta in a region between the segmental vessels. This tissue will contain the thoracic duct, and it may be ligated en masse using a heavy ligature (e.g., 0 silk), and then divided with the vessel sealer or curved monopolar scissors.

- Dissect along the posterior mediastinum and dissect the thoracic duct en bloc with the esophagus (optional).
  - At this point, the esophagus has been circumferentially mobilized at the hiatus.

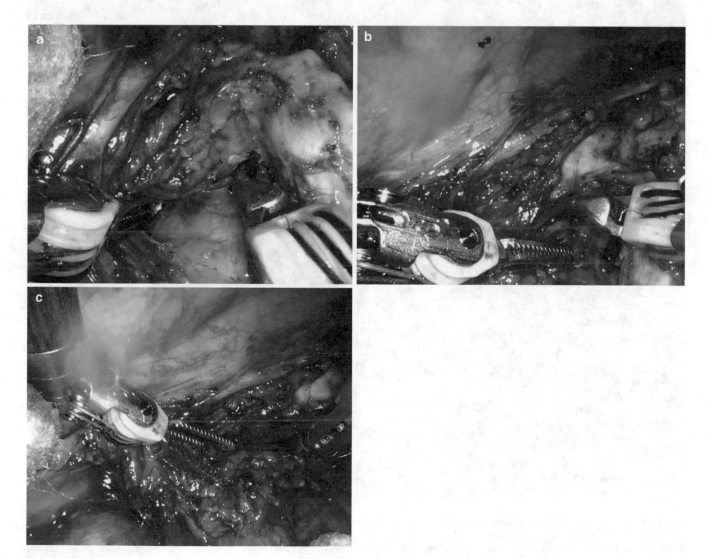

Fig. 4.14 (**a**) A subcarinal nodal dissection is performed using bipolar electrocautery. (**b**) The left main bronchus is identified, and the posterior vascular supply to the node is carefully divided. (**c**) The vessels entering the subcarinal node at the carina are divided, and the node is removed

– Divide the remaining attachments to posterior mediastinum with the vessel sealer from inferior to superior, retracting the esophagus and surrounding tissue laterally and anteriorly. The plane of dissection is adjacent to the vertebral bodies, aorta, pericardium, and left main bronchus (Fig. 4.15c).

Mobilization and Division of the Esophagus

• Mobilize the esophagus above the level of the carina to an extent that depends on the location of the tumor and the site of the planned anastomosis.
  – As dissection proceeds more cephalad along the posterior membranous trachea, the plane of dissection should be adjacent to the esophageal wall to avoid injury to either the left recurrent laryngeal nerve or the membranous airway. Bipolar electrocautery is useful to prevent heat transfer to the membranous airway (Fig. 4.15d).
• Divide the right vagus nerve at the level of the distal trachea.
• Mobilize at least 4 cm of esophagus away from the airway and surrounding tissue to allow creation of a tension-free anastomosis. Bipolar electrocautery should be used to prevent airway injury.
  – Ensure that the nasogastric tube has been withdrawn above the level of planned transection.
  – Divide the esophagus using a robot linear stapler (SureForm™ 60 instrument, green 4.3 mm load).

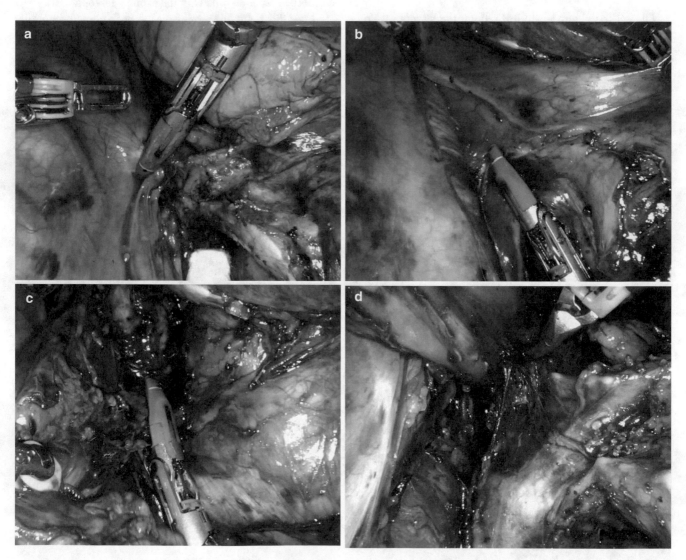

Fig. 4.15 (a) The subcarinal nodal tissue has been resected, and the posterior pleura is opened along the course of the azygos vein. The thoracic duct may be taken either en bloc with the specimen or left intact. (b) Further posterior dissection proceeds from inferior to superior along the anterior aspect of the descending thoracic aorta. (c) The posterior attachments to the pericardium are divided to the level of the left main bronchus. (d) The esophagus is elevated off the membranous airway to above the level of the azygos vein using bipolar electrocautery

Conduit Delivery and Specimen Extraction

- Retract the esophageal specimen cephalad and deliver the attached conduit into the lower chest (Fig. 4.16).
- Disconnect the specimen from the conduit.
  - Either extracted by enlarging the anterior 8th interspace port (Arm 3) or left detached in the anterior chest and extracted at the end of the case which allows maintenance of CO_2 insufflation and preservation of exposure (my preference).
  - Extraction should be performed by creating a 4–5 cm incision at the site of the 12 mm port and placing a wound protector prior to removing the specimen.
- Deliver the conduit further into the chest.
  - Care should be taken to ensure that the conduit is not twisted. The staple line of the conduit should lie laterally (i.e., at 12 o'clock position to the plane of the bed).

- There is no haptic feedback with the robot, so it is very important to use gentle retraction as serosal tears may easily occur as one tries to pull the conduit into the chest (Fig. 4.16b).
- Judging when all the conduit has been delivered can be difficult sometimes. However, if one is able to visualize the beginning of the lesser curvature staple line on the antrum of the stomach, usually the pylorus will be at the level of the hiatus.
- If an assistant port has been placed, the bedside assistant can sometimes get a better sense of tension on the conduit and help in gentle traction with a 5 mm thoracoscopic grasper.
- The attached omental flap should be fully delivered into the chest by gently teasing it up as it can sometimes ball up in the abdomen and prevent the conduit from being delivered further.

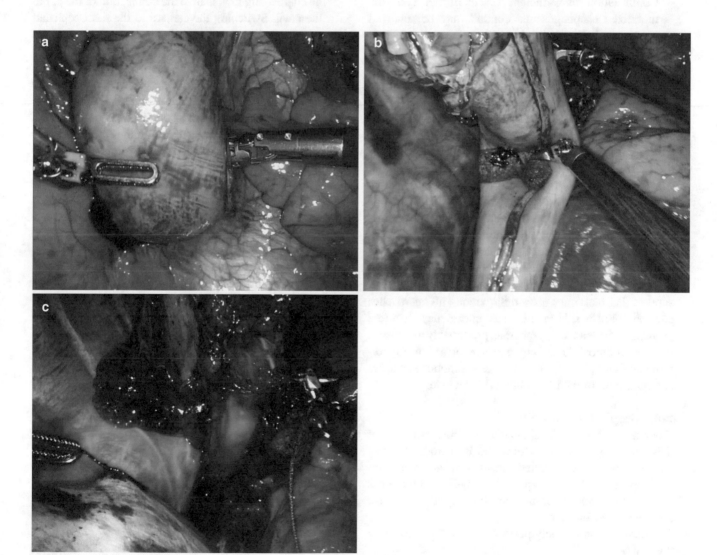

Fig. 4.16 (**a**) The esophagus is retracted cephalad which pulls the attached conduit through the hiatus and into the chest, elevated off the membranous airway to above the level of the azygos vein using bipolar electrocautery. (**b**) Using blunt retraction, the conduit is pulled fully into the chest, and the site of potential anastomosis is determined. (**c**) Additional ICG (12.5 mg) is administered intravenously to assess the perfusion of the mobilized esophagus as well as the conduit

- Place the conduit adjacent to the divided proximal esophagus under gentle tension.
- Identify the site of anastomosis.
  - The anastomosis should be placed on the most well-vascularized part of the conduit, which is typically on the greater curvature.
  - Placement of the anastomosis on the anterior wall of the stomach potentially risks creating a hypo-perfused region between the gastric staple line and the lateral aspect of the anastomosis; however, it is not known whether this has any clinical consequences, and many surgeons routinely place the anastomosis on the anterior conduit without negative effect.
  - A novel technique of siting the anastomosis right along the previous gastric staple line has recently been described and with excellent outcomes, which might have a useful application for the robotic approach [13, 15].
  - Confirmation of sufficient vascularity of both the mobilized esophagus and conduit may be achieved using near-infrared imaging and intravenous injection of ICG (Fig. 4.16c).

Intrathoracic Anastomosis

- As with open transthoracic esophagectomy, there are several different ways to perform the anastomosis, arguably the most critical aspect to the entire procedure, and no consensus exists as to which is the best method. Factors that influence the decision of which technique to use include whether a skilled bedside assistant is available, degree of technical expertise required, site of anastomosis, and, to a large extent, tradition. Comparative data regarding anastomotic technique are mainly retrospective and somewhat limited; however, there is some evidence to support that leak rates are similar among all approaches and that a linear side-to-side anastomosis may have less propensity to lead to dysphagia, presumably because a wider anastomosis is less prone to develop a clinically relevant stricture [16–21]. The three anastomotic techniques commonly performed for robotic ILE include:

Circular Stapled Anastomosis

- The benefit of a circular stapled anastomosis (CS) is that it is relatively easy to perform and is reproducible [5]. However, it requires a skilled bedside assistant to position and deploy the device. Typically, a 25–29 mm stapler is used, which can sometimes be challenging to traverse narrow intercostal spaces.
- There are two commonly performed method of securing the anvil.
  - The anvil is passed into the chest through the access incision and placed into the lumen of the divided esophagus [22, 23]. A purse-string suture (e.g., 3-0 Prolene) is then placed, taking full-thickness bites of

tissue including the muscle wall and the mucosa, in either a running baseball or horizontal mattress fashion, and tied down around the stem of the anvil. An additional purse string is sometimes placed to ensure close approximation of all tissue within the stapler.
  - The second method utilizes the use of the DST Series™ EEA™ OrVil™ device (Covidien, Dublin, Ireland) which is delivered perorally [24]. The stapled end of the esophagus is incised either in the middle of the staple line or at one end of it, and the nasogastric tube portion of the OrVil™ is brought out through the defect. The stem of the OrVil™ anvil is then delivered and the NG removed.
- The conduit is then delivered into the chest, a gastrotomy of sufficient length is made in the tip of the conduit and the stapler device placed into the conduit, and the pin is brought out on the greater curvature of the stomach.
  - Often, the anastomosis is in the upper chest, and it may be challenging to visualize the connection of the pin to the anvil. Switching the camera to the most cephalad port (Arm 4) and use of a 30-degree camera may help in this regard.
- Once the pin and anvil are connected, the stapler is closed, taking care that no unwanted tissue has crept into the space between the stomach and esophagus, and the stapler is fired, creating an end to side anastomosis.
- The stapler is withdrawn, and the circular pieces of transected stomach and esophagus are examined to ensure that they are circumferentially intact.
- The nasogastric tube is then guided from the esophagus and into the distal conduit. Redundant conduit is divided using a robotic linear stapler. The anastomosis and proximal conduit staple line may be buttressed with Lembert sutures (e.g., 2-0 silk).

Hand-Sewn Anastomosis

- This is the most technically challenging and labor-intensive method of creating the anastomosis; however, it is very flexible and particularly useful for high intrathoracic anastomoses or if there is insufficient length on the gastric tube as an end-to-end anastomosis may be created at the tip of the conduit.
  - A bedside assistant is not critical as the entire anastomosis is performed by the console surgeon.
- Techniques vary; however, most commonly, a two-layered anastomosis is performed [25, 26].
- The site of the anastomosis may be on the posterior (harder) or anterior (easier) aspect of the stomach tube.
- Place a backrow of interrupted sutures (e.g., 2-0 silk) between the muscle wall of the esophagus and the serosa of the stomach.
- Create a gastrotomy, and place a running, full-thickness stitch between the esophagus and gastric conduit.
  - It is often easiest to start two separate suture lines, which then meet anteriorly at the completion of the anastomosis and may be tied together.

– Maintaining traction on the suture material is imperative, and barbed sutures are very useful in this regard, e.g., V-Loc™ (Covidien, Dublin, Ireland) or STRATAFIX™ (Johnson & Johnson, New Brunswick, New Jersey). An anterior row of Lembert sutures, e.g., 2-0 silk, is then placed.

Linear Stapled (Modified Collard) Anastomosis

• The benefits of this approach include the fact that it is a wide anastomosis and less prone to stricture formation, can be performed completely robotically without a bed-side assistant, and avoids having to place a posterior line of sutures so is slightly quicker than a completely hand-sewn technique (Fig. 4.17).

• I typically place the anastomosis on the posterior aspect of the stomach, though the anterior surface is certainly easier and arguably has similar results.

• Select a point on the greater curvature of the stomach that represents the maximal extent of the anastomosis.

– Suture this region to the proximal underside of the mobilized esophagus (Fig. 4.18a).

• The esophagus is divided using a linear robotic stapler ensuring that at least 4–5 cm of esophagus have been mobilized (Fig. 4.18b, c). The staple line is removed using the monopolar scissors (Fig. 4.18d). The esophagus is then extended along the posterior wall of the conduit and a small gastrostomy made (Fig. 4.18e). A full-thickness suture is placed connecting the esophagus to the stomach at the midpoint of the gastrostomy, keeping the suture ends long so that they may be used for retraction (Fig. 4.18f).

• A 60 mm linear robotic stapler is advanced into the two lumens, with the cartridge being placed in the stomach and the anvil in the esophagus (Fig. 4.19a). The retraction suture is used to pull the esophagus and stomach into the stapler jaws. A 45 mm stapled common posterior wall is created (Fig. 4.19b). The anterior defect is then closed in

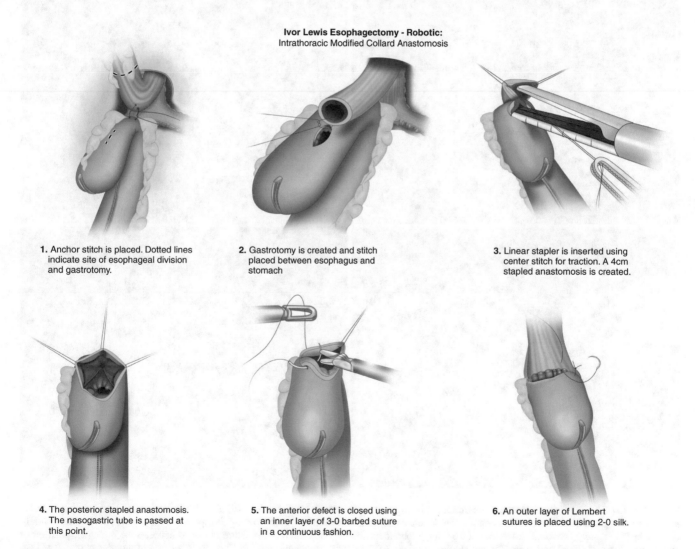

Ivor Lewis Esophagectomy - Robotic:
Intrathoracic Modified Collard Anastomosis

1. Anchor stitch is placed. Dotted lines indicate site of esophageal division and gastrotomy.

2. Gastrotomy is created and stitch placed between esophagus and stomach

3. Linear stapler is inserted using center stitch for traction. A 4cm stapled anastomosis is created.

4. The posterior stapled anastomosis. The nasogastric tube is passed at this point.

5. The anterior defect is closed using an inner layer of 3-0 barbed suture in a continuous fashion.

6. An outer layer of Lembert sutures is placed using 2-0 silk.

Fig. 4.17 Modified collard anastomosis. (**a**) An anchor stitch is placed between the esophagus and conduit. Dotted lines indicate the site of division of the esophagus and the gastrotomy. (**b**) Gastrotomy is created and stitch placed between esophagus and stomach. (**c**) Linear stapler is inserted using center stitch for traction. A 4 cm stapled anastomosis is created. (**d**) The posterior stapled anastomosis. The nasogastric tube is passed at this point. (**e**) The anterior defect is closed using an inner layer of 3-0 barbed suture in a continuous fashion. (**f**) An outer layer of Lembert sutures is placed using 2-0 silk

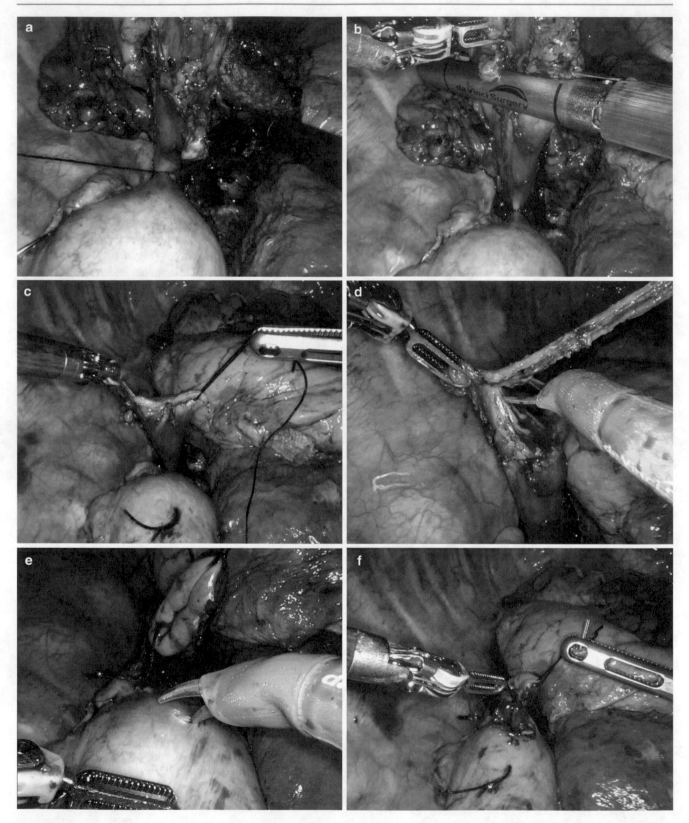

Fig. 4.18 (**a**) The posterior aspect of the mobilized esophagus is sutured to the greater curvature of the conduit. (**b**) The esophagus is divided approximately 4–5 cm distal to the suture using a robotic linear stapler with 3.5 mm (blue) or 4.3 mm (green) staple cartridges. (**c**) The divided esophagus sutured at its deeper aspect to the greater curve of the conduit. The stitch on the conduit represents the distal extent of the malperfused conduit. (**d**) The staple line on the divided esophagus is excised. (**e**) A gastrotomy is created on the greater curve of the conduit. (**f**) A full-thickness suture is placed between the 6 o'clock position of the esophagus and the 12 o'clock position of the gastrotomy. It is kept long to aid in retraction while the stapler is placed

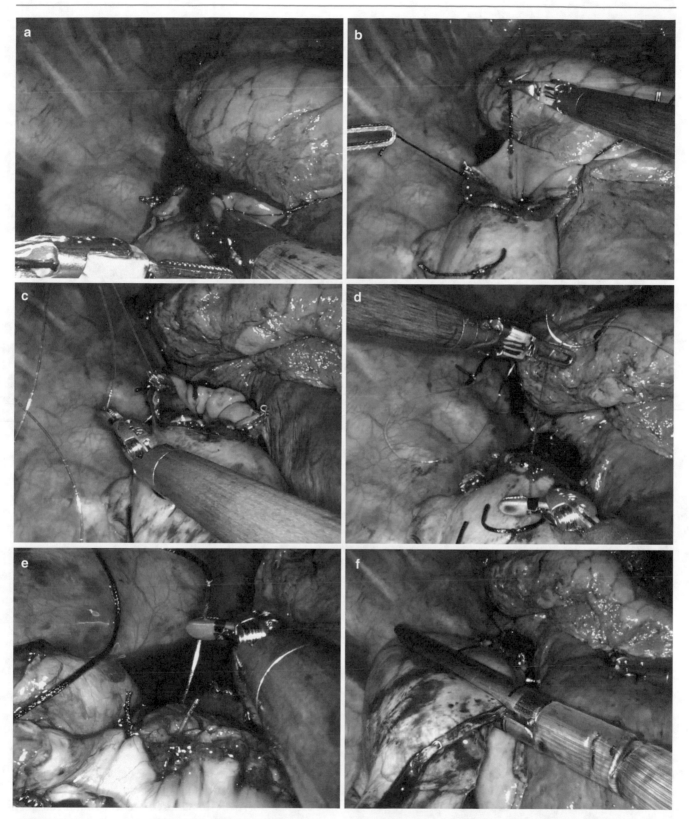

Fig. 4.19 (**a**) A linear robotic stapler (Arm 3) with 3.5 mm (blue) staple cartridge is passed so that the cartridge is in the stomach and the anvil in the esophageal lumen. The retraction stitch helps pull the tissue into the jaws of the stapler. The stapler is advanced to 40 mm. (**b**) The posterior stapled anastomosis is completed. The nasogastric tube is passed across the anastomosis and carefully guided into the conduit. (**c**) The defect is closed in two layers using a full-thickness inner layer of 3-0 barbed suture. (**d**) Two sutures are used beginning at each end and meeting in the middle. (**e**) An outer layer of 2-0 silk Lembert sutures is placed. (**f**) Redundant (malperfused) conduit is excised with a robotic linear stapler and the staple line oversewn with 2-0 silk Lembert sutures

two layers as described above for a hand-sewn anastomosis (Fig. 4.19c–e). Redundant conduit is excised, and the remaining conduit is sutured to overlap and reinforce the anastomosis (Fig. 4.19f).

Flap Coverage, Drain Placement, and the Hiatal Defect

- Position the omental flap between the conduit and the airway, and wrap circumferentially around the anastomosis (Fig. 4.20a). Secured it at multiple points with suture so that it does not become dislodged (Fig. 4.20b).

- If the left pleural space has been entered, a drain is placed posterior to the conduit, across the mediastinum, and into the left pleural space (e.g., 19 Fr Blake). Alternatively, this may be placed at the time of the abdominal phase and brought out through the left subcostal port site.
- Place a drain alongside the conduit in the ipsilateral posterior pleural space (e.g., 24 Fr Argyle).
- Examine the hiatus, and suture the conduit circumferentially to the left and right crus (Fig. 4.21).
  - This prevents cephalad migration of any redundant intra-abdominal conduit into the chest, which may interfere with conduit emptying, and potentially less-

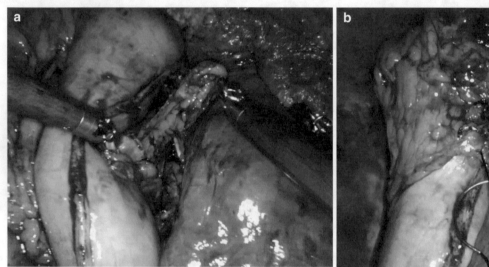
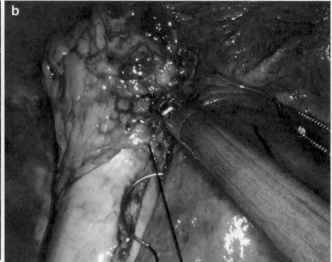

Fig. 4.20 (**a**) The omental flap is placed between the conduit and the airway and wrapped around the anastomosis. (**b**) The omental flap circumferentially covering the anastomosis and separating the conduit away from the airway

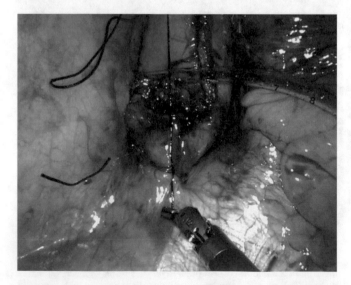

Fig. 4.21 The conduit is sutured to the left and right crus to prevent herniation of the conduit or abdominal viscera

ens the risk of herniation of abdominal contents into either pleural cavity, which is a phenomenon that appears to be much more frequent after minimally invasive esophagectomy than it is with open procedures [27, 28].

Postoperative Management (Table 4.1)

- Patients are extubated in the operating room and brought to the postanesthesia care unit for initial recovery. The intensive care unit is not utilized. Patients are then transferred to a thoracic surgery telemetry unit with continuous EKG and pulse oximetry monitoring.
- Activity – Out of bed to chair on postoperative day 0 (POD 0). Thereafter, ambulate at least four times daily.

Table 4.1 Perioperative management of patients undergoing robotic-assisted Ivor Lewis esophagectomy

	Day of surgery (POD 0)	POD 1 discharge	Post-discharge
Drain management	Silicone NGT placed intraoperatively	Low continuous suction until POD 3. Removed POD 4 (or when volume <400 cc/24 hour)	None
	24 Fr Argyle, right chest; 19 Fr Blake left chest if left pleural space entered	Negative 20 cm H$_2$O suction. Removed day after commencement of oral liquids (usually POD 5) if no evidence of anastomotic leak	None
	Foley catheter. I/O q1h for 12 hours	Remove Foley catheter – POD 2	None
	A-line	Remove A-line – POD 1	None
Diet	Clear liquid diet up until 2 hours before check-in time	NPO	Full liquid diet
		Esophagogram when NGT removed, usually POD 4. Oral liquids started if negative for leak	Esophagogram (POD 10–14). Soft diet started if negative for leak
Pain management	*In pre-op*:	*NPO*:	*Discharge*:
	Celebrex 200 mg PO; tramadol 300 mg PO; gabapentin 300 mg PO	Acetaminophen 1 gram IVPB q6h; Toradol 15 mg IV q6h; Dilaudid 0.5 mg IV every 3–4 hours prn pain or PCA	Acetaminophen 1 gram PO q6h × 10 days; Celebrex 200 mg PO BID × 10 days; gabapentin taper of 300 mg PO q8h × 7 days, then 300 mg PO q12h × 7 days, then 300 mg PO daily × 7 days (total 42 capsules or 260 mL elixir)
	Intra-op:	*After PO intake began*:	
	Liposomal bupivacaine 1.3%	Acetaminophen 1 gram PO q6h; Celebrex 200 mg PO BID; gabapentin 300 mg PO q8h	Seven-day supply of opiate for breakthrough pain according to patient's opioid requirements during hospitalization
		Initiate oral opiates as clinically appropriate for breakthrough pain	
	POD 0:	*Adjuvant therapy*	
	Acetaminophen 1 gram IVPB q6h; Toradol 15 mg IV q6h; Dilaudid 0.5 mg IV q3–4 hours	Consider Robaxin 500–750 mg IV q8h (avoid IV with renal dysfunction)	Adjuvant analgesics as needed
	May initiate PCA if needed (persistent pain score ≥4)	Consider Lidoderm patch (may have one to three patches to chest wall)	
		Consider ice therapy	
VTE prophylaxis	Heparin 5000 units subcutaneous >30mins pre-incision	Heparin 5000 units subcutaneous q8h	Consider daily Lovenox injections for first 30 days post-op on discharge based on Caprini score ≥9

- Venous thromboembolism precautions – Heparin 5000 units q8 hours while inpatient. Daily Lovenox for the first 30 days postoperatively if Caprini score ≥9.
- Analgesia – POD 0 to 4 – acetaminophen 1 g i.v. q6h, ketorolac 15 mg i.v. q6h, hydromorphone 0.5 mg i.v. q3–4 h PRN. May initiate patient-controlled analgesia (PCA) hydromorphone if needed. POD 4, if taking oral liquids – acetaminophen 1 g po q6h, celecoxib 200 mg po q12h, gabapentin 300 mg po q8h.
- Drain and nutritional management – Nasogastric tube to low intermittent suction until POD 4. Removed if daily volume <400 cc and no conduit dilatation on CXR. Esophagogram on POD 4. Begin clear liquids if no evidence of leak. Advance to full liquids on POD 5. Chest drain removed on POD 5 if no evidence of leak. Patients remain on full liquid diet for 7–10 days before repeat esophagogram. If no evidence of leak, advanced to post-

gastrectomy diet. Urinary catheter typically removed on POD 2.

Outcomes of Robot-Assisted Ivor Lewis Esophagectomy

The majority of centers performing ILER currently use a totally robotic approach. In the reported literature, approximately 70% of patients receive preoperative chemotherapy or chemoradiation treatment. The most common anastomotic technique is a circular stapled anastomosis, with at least four centers utilizing the OrVil™ device (Covidien, Dublin, Ireland) (Table 4.2). The weighted mean operative time of the 18 series reported in Table 4.1 is 389 minutes (range 304–661 minutes) with a conversion rate of only 4% (range 0–21%).

Node harvesting appears to be excellent with studies reporting that on average, 22 nodes were resected, and 97% of patients had R0 resection. Operative mortality is low, at 1.3%, and reported morbidity ranges between 19% and 79% (weighted mean 39%) (Table 4.3). Anastomotic leaks are comparable to what has been reported for open procedures, at 8%, but there is wide variation across studies ranging from as low as 3% to as high as 21%, though not all leaks have required intervention. Mean length of hospitalization in these studies is 10 days. Overall, therefore, robotic-assisted Ivor Lewis esophagectomy has been demonstrated to be feasible and appears to have an excellent safety profile while providing adequate oncologic treatment. Conversion rates are quite low compared to what has been reported for traditional MIE [29, 30].

Table 4.2 Robotic-assisted Ivor Lewis esophagectomy, operative approach

Author, year	Center	n	Abdominal phase	Thoracic phase	Anastomosis	Operative time (mins)
Cerfolio, 2013 [26]	Alabama, USA	22	L	R	HS(16), LS (6)	367
De la Fuente, 2013 [31]	Orlando, USA	50	R	R	CS (OrVil™)	445
Hernandez, 2013 [32]	Tallahassee, USA	52	R	R	CS (OrVil™)	442
Trugeda, 2014 [33]	Cantabria, Spain	14	R	R	HS(16), LS (6)	NR
Abbott, 2015 [34]	Madison, USA	134	R	R	NR	407
Hodari, 2015 [35]	Detroit, USA	54	L	R	LS	368
Sarkaria, 2016 [36] §	New York, USA	100	R	R	CS	379
Amaral, 2017 [24]	Tampa, USA	237	R	R	CS (OrVil™)	364
Egberts, 2017 [25]	Keil, Germany	75	R	R	HS	392
Okusanya, 2017 [37]	Pittsburg, USA	24	R	R	CS	661
Wang, 2019 [38] *	Chengdu, China	31	R	R	CS	387
Sarkaria, 2019 [39] §	New York, USA	64	R	R	CS	384
Tagkalos, 2019	Mainz, Germany	50	R	R	CS	383
Wang, 2019 [40] *	Chengdu, China	37	R	R	LS	340
Zhang, 2019 [21] *	Chengdu, China	77	R	R	CS(42), LS (35)	343–356
Zhang, 2019 [41]	Shanghai, China	76	R	R	CS(40), HS (36)	304
Meredith, 2020 [29]	Tallahassee, USA	144	R	R	CS (OrVil™)	409
Van der Sluis, 2020 [42]	Mainz, Germany	100	R	R	CS	415

§ possible duplication of patients, * possible duplication of patients, *R* robotic, *L* laparoscopic, *HS* hand sewn, *CS* circular stapled, *LS* linear stapled, *NR* not reported

Table 4.3 Robotic-assisted Ivor Lewis esophagectomy, outcomes

Author, year	Conversion	Leak	LOS	Morbidity	Mortality	# nodes resected	R0 rate (%)
Cerfolio, 2013 [26]	5%	9%	7	36%	0%	18	100%
De la Fuente, 2013 [31]	0%	4%	9	28%	0%	19	100%
Hernandez, 2013 [32]	0%	4%	NR	27%	0%	19	NR
Trugeda, 2014 [33]	0%	21%	13	43%	0%	18	100%
Abbott, 2015 [34]	0%	4%	10	27%	2%	NR	100%
Hodari, 2015 [35]	0%	6%	13	NR	2%	16	100%
Sarkaria, 2016 [36] §	10%	6%	9	52%	0%	24	90%
Amaral, 2017 [24]	NR	15%	9	48%	3%	21	NR
Egberts, 2017 [25]	21%	16%	16	73% (90d)	4%	29	96%
Okusanya, 2017 [37]	8%	4%	8	68%	0%	26	96%
Wang, 2019 [38] *	0%	6%	12	19%	0%	17	97%
Sarkaria, 2019 [39] §	NR	3%	9	39%	2%	25	97%
Tagkalos, 2019	NR	12%	12	NR	0%	27	92%
Wang, 2019 [40] *	NR	8%	10	NR	0%	NR	100%
Zhang, 2019 [21] *	3%	6%	12	NR	0%	21–23	100%
Zhang, 2019 [41]	3%	9%	9	32%	0%	18	100%
Meredith, 2020 [29]	0%	3%	9	24%	1%	20	100%
Van der Sluis, 2020 [42]	2%	8%	11	30%	1%	29	92%

§ possible duplication of patients, * possible duplication of patients, *NR* not reported, *LOS* length of stay (median, days)

References

1. Ferlay J, Ervik M, Lam F, Colombet M, Mery L, Pineros M, et al. Global cancer observatory. Lyon: International Agency for Research on Cancer; 2018. Available from: https://gco.iarc.fr/today

2. Arnold M, Laversanne M, Brown LM, Devesa SS, Bray F. Predicting the future burden of esophageal cancer by histological subtype: international trends in incidence up to 2030. Am J Gastroenterol. 2017;112(8):1247–55.

3. Haverkamp L, Seesing MF, Ruurda JP, Boone J, Hillegersberg RV. Worldwide trends in surgical techniques in the treatment of esophageal and gastroesophageal junction cancer. Dis Esophagus. 2017;30(1):1–7.

4. Cerfolio RJ, Laliberte AS, Blackmon S, Ruurda JP, van Hillegersberg R, Sarkaria I, et al. Minimally invasive esophagectomy: a consensus statement. Ann Thorac Surg. 2020;110(4):1417–26.

5. Egberts JH, Biebl M, Perez DR, Mees ST, Grimminger PP, Muller-Stich BP, et al. Robot-assisted oesophagectomy: recommendations towards a standardised Ivor Lewis procedure. J Gastrointest Surg. 2019;23(7):1485–92. https://doi.org/10.1007/s11605-019-04207-y. Epub 2019 Apr 1.

6. Sarkaria IS, Bains MS, Finley DJ, Adusumilli PS, Huang J, Rusch VW, et al. Intraoperative near-infrared fluorescence imaging as an adjunct to robotic-assisted minimally invasive esophagectomy. Innovations (Phila). 2014;9(5):391–3. https://doi.org/10.1097/IMI.0000000000000091.

7. Nobel T, Tan KS, Barbetta A, Adusumilli P, Bains M, Bott M, et al. Does pyloric drainage have a role in the era of minimally invasive esophagectomy? Surg Endosc. 2019;33(10):3218–27.

8. Antonoff MB, Puri V, Meyers BF, Baumgartner K, Bell JM, Broderick S, et al. Comparison of pyloric intervention strategies at the time of esophagectomy: is more better? Ann Thorac Surg. 2014;97(6):1950–7. discussion 657-8.

9. Marchese S, Qureshi YA, Hafiz SP, Dawas K, Turner P, Mughal MM, et al. Intraoperative pyloric interventions during oesophagectomy: a multicentre study. J Gastrointest Surg. 2018;22(8):1319–24.

10. Arya S, Markar SR, Karthikesalingam A, Hanna GB. The impact of pyloric drainage on clinical outcome following esophagectomy: a systematic review. Dis Esophagus. 2015;28(4):326–35.

11. Cerfolio RJ, Bryant AS, Canon CL, Dhawan R, Eloubeidi MA. Is botulinum toxin injection of the pylorus during Ivor Lewis [corrected] esophagogastrectomy the optimal drainage strategy? J Thorac Cardiovasc Surg. 2009;137(3):565–72.

12. Eldaif SM, Lee R, Adams KN, Kilgo PD, Gruszynski MA, Force SD, et al. Intrapyloric botulinum injection increases postoperative esophagectomy complications. Ann Thorac Surg. 2014;97(6):1959–64. discussion 64-5.

13. Kesler KA, Ramchandani NK, Jalal SI, Stokes SM, Mankins MR, Ceppa D, et al. Outcomes of a novel intrathoracic esophagogastric anastomotic technique. J Thorac Cardiovasc Surg. 2018;156(4):1739–45 e1.

14. van Boxel GI, Kingma BF, Voskens FJ, Ruurda JP, van Hillegersberg R. Robotic-assisted minimally invasive esophagectomy: past, present and future. J Thorac Dis. 2020;12(2):54 62. https://doi.org/10.21037/jtd.2019.06.75.

15. Hagen JA. A novel intrathoracic esophagogastric anastomotic technique: potential benefit for patients undergoing a robotic-assisted minimally invasive esophagectomy. J Thorac Cardiovasc Surg. 2018;156(4):1746–7. https://doi.org/10.1016/j.jtcvs.2018.05.116. Epub Jun 23.

16. Price TN, Nichols FC, Harmsen WS, Allen MS, Cassivi SD, Wigle DA, et al. A comprehensive review of anastomotic technique in 432 esophagectomies. Ann Thorac Surg. 2013;95(4):1154–60. discussion 60-1.

17. Blackmon SH, Correa AM, Wynn B, Hofstetter WL, Martin LW, Mehran RJ, et al. Propensity-matched analysis of three techniques for intrathoracic esophagogastric anastomosis. Ann Thorac Surg. 2007;83(5):1805–13. discussion 13.

18. Law S, Fok M, Chu KM, Wong J. Comparison of hand-sewn and stapled esophagogastric anastomosis after esophageal resection for cancer: a prospective randomized controlled trial. Ann Surg. 1997;226(2):169–73.

19. Deng XF, Liu QX, Zhou D, Min JX, Dai JG. Hand-sewn vs linearly stapled esophagogastric anastomosis for esophageal cancer: a meta-analysis. World J Gastroenterol. 2015;21(15):4757–64.

20. Plat VD, Stam WT, Schoonmade LJ, Heineman DJ, van der Peet DL, Daams F. Implementation of robot-assisted Ivor Lewis procedure: robotic hand-sewn, linear or circular technique? Am J Surg. 2019;26(19):31545–4.

21. Zhang H, Wang Z, Zheng Y, Geng Y, Wang F, Chen LQ, et al. Robotic side-to-side and end-to-side stapled esophagogastric anastomosis of Ivor Lewis esophagectomy for cancer. World J Surg. 2019;43(12):3074–82. https://doi.org/10.1007/s00268-019-5133-5.

22. Sarkaria IS, Rizk NP. Robotic-assisted minimally invasive esophagectomy: the Ivor Lewis approach. Thorac Surg Clin. 2014;24(2):211–22.

23. Grimminger PP, Hadzijusufovic E, Babic B, van der Sluis PC, Lang H. Innovative fully robotic 4-arm Ivor Lewis esophagectomy for esophageal cancer (RAMIE4). Dis Esophagus. 2020;33(3). (pii):5450338. https://doi.org/10.1093/dote/doz015.

24. Amaral M, Pimiento J, Fontaine JP. Robotic esophagectomy: the Moffitt Cancer Center experience. Ann Cardiothorac Surg. 2017;6(2):186–9. https://doi.org/10.21037/acs.2017.03.21.

25. Egberts JH, Stein H, Aselmann H, Hendricks A, Becker T. Fully robotic da Vinci Ivor-Lewis esophagectomy in four-arm technique-problems and solutions. Dis Esophagus. 2017;30(12):1–9. https://doi.org/10.1093/dote/dox098.

26. Cerfolio RJ, Wei B, Hawn MT, Minnich DJ. Robotic esophagectomy for cancer: early results and lessons learned. Semin Thorac Cardiovasc Surg. 2016;28(1):160–9.

27. Gooszen JAH, Slaman AE, van Dieren S, Gisbertz SS, van Berge Henegouwen MI. Incidence and treatment of symptomatic diaphragmatic hernia after esophagectomy for cancer. Ann Thorac Surg. 2018;106(1):199–206.

28. Gust L, Nafteux P, Allemann P, Tuech JJ, El Nakadi I, Collet D, et al. Hiatal hernia after oesophagectomy: a large European survey. Eur J Cardiothorac Surg. 2019;55(6):1104–12.

29. de la Fuente SG, Weber J, Hoffe SE, Shridhar R, Karl R, Meredith KL. Initial experience from a large referral center with robotic-assisted Ivor Lewis esophagogastrectomy for oncologic purposes. Surg Endosc. 2013;27(9):3339–47.

30. Hernandez JM, Dimou F, Weber J, Almhanna K, Hoffe S, Shridhar R, et al. Defining the learning curve for robotic-assisted esophagogastrectomy. J Gastrointest Surg. 2013;17(8):1346–51.

31. Trugeda S, Fernandez-Diaz MJ, Rodriguez-Sanjuan JC, Palazuelos CM, Fernandez-Escalante C, Gomez-Fleitas M. Initial results of robot-assisted Ivor-Lewis oesophagectomy with intrathoracic hand-sewn anastomosis in the prone position. Int J Med Robot. 2014;10(4):397–403. https://doi.org/10.1002/rcs.587. Epub 2014 Apr 29.

32. Abbott A, Shridhar R, Hoffe S, Almhanna K, Doepker M, Saeed N, et al. Robotic assisted Ivor Lewis esophagectomy in the elderly patient. J Gastrointest Oncol. 2015;6(1):31–8.

33. Hodari A, Park KU, Lace B, Tsiouris A, Hammoud Z. Robot-assisted minimally invasive Ivor Lewis esophagectomy with real-time perfusion assessment. Ann Thorac Surg. 2015;100(3):947–52. https://doi.org/10.1016/j.athoracsur.2015.03.084. Epub Jun 24.

34. Sarkaria IS, Rizk NP, Grosser R, Goldman D, Finley DJ, Ghanie A, et al. Attaining proficiency in robotic-assisted minimally invasive esophagectomy while maximizing safety during procedure development. Innovations (Phila). 2016;11(4):268–73.

35. Okusanya OT, Sarkaria IS, Hess NR, Nason KS, Sanchez MV, Levy RM, et al. Robotic assisted minimally invasive esophagec-

tomy (RAMIE): the University of Pittsburgh Medical Center initial experience. Ann Cardiothorac Surg. 2017;6(2):179–85. https://doi.org/10.21037/acs.2017.03.12.

36. Wang WP, Chen LQ, Zhang HL, Yang YS, He SL, Yuan Y, et al. Modified intrathoracic esophagogastrostomy with minimally invasive robot-assisted Ivor-Lewis esophagectomy for cancer. Dig Surg. 2019;36(3):218–25. https://doi.org/10.1159/000495361. Epub 2018 Dec 5.

37. Sarkaria IS, Rizk NP, Goldman DA, Sima C, Tan KS, Bains MS, et al. Early quality of life outcomes after robotic-assisted minimally invasive and open esophagectomy. Ann Thorac Surg. 2019;108(3):920–8. https://doi.org/10.1016/j.athoracsur.2018.11.075. Epub 9 Apr 23.

38. Wang F, Zhang H, Zheng Y, Wang Z, Geng Y, Wang Y. Intrathoracic side-to-side esophagogastrostomy with a linear stapler and barbed suture in robot-assisted Ivor Lewis esophagectomy. J Surg Oncol. 2019;120(7):1142–7. https://doi.org/10.1002/jso.25698. Epub 2019 Sep 18.

39. van der Sluis PC, Tagkalos E, Hadzijusufovic E, Babic B, Uzun E, van Hillegersberg R, et al. Robot-assisted minimally invasive esophagectomy with intrathoracic anastomosis (Ivor Lewis): promising results in 100 consecutive patients (the European experience). J Gastrointest Surg. 2020;18(10):019–04510.

40. Zhang Y, Han Y, Gan Q, Xiang J, Jin R, Chen K, et al. Early outcomes of robot-assisted versus thoracoscopic-assisted Ivor Lewis esophagectomy for esophageal cancer: a propensity score-matched study. Ann Surg Oncol. 2019;26(5):1284–91. https://doi.org/10.1245/s10434-019-07273-3. Epub 2019 Mar 6.

41. Meredith K, Blinn P, Maramara T, Takahashi C, Huston J, Shridhar R. Comparative outcomes of minimally invasive and robotic-assisted esophagectomy. Surg Endosc. 2020;34(2):814–20. https://doi.org/10.1007/s00464-019-6834-7. Epub 2019 Jun 10.

42. Halpern AL, Friedman C, Torphy RJ, Al-Musawi MH, Mitchell JD, Scott CD, et al. Conversion to open surgery during minimally invasive esophagectomy portends worse short-term outcomes: an analysis of the National Cancer Database. Surg Endosc. 2019;7(10):019–07124.

Robot-Assisted McKeown Esophagectomy

Min P. Kim

Three-hole esophagectomy or McKeown esophagectomy can be performed using the robot. We reserve this approach for patients with a mid esophageal tumor where the anastomosis in the neck allows complete resection of the tumor with negative surgical margins. Typically, patients with locally advanced esophageal cancer undergo induction chemoradiation therapy. Afterward, the patient undergoes restaging with PET-CT and EUS. Patients with concern for the invasion of the airway on the imaging or on EUS, they undergo flexible bronchoscopy with EBUS to ensure there is no invasion of the trachea. Patients also undergo a cardiac and pulmonary evaluation to ensure that patient is a good candidate for surgical treatment.

Equipment

- AirSeal (ConMED, Utica, NY)
- Xi Robot
  - Cadiere Forceps (Intuitive Surgical, Sunnyvale, CA)
  - Tip-Up Fenestrated Grasper (Intuitive Surgical, Sunnyvale, CA)
  - Mega SutureCut Needle Driver (Intuitive Surgical, Sunnyvale, CA)
  - Long Bipolar Grasper (Intuitive Surgical, Sunnyvale, CA)
  - Vessel sealer (Intuitive Surgical, Sunnyvale, CA)
  - EndoWrist Stapler (Intuitive Surgical, Sunnyvale, CA)

Electronic supplementary material The online version of this chapter (https://doi.org/10.1007/978-3-030-55669-3_5) contains supplementary material, which is available to authorized users.

M. P. Kim (✉)
Division of Thoracic Surgery, Department of Surgery and Cardiothoracic Surgery, Weill Cornell Medical College Department of Surgery, Houston Methodist Hospital, Houston, TX, USA
e-mail: mpkim@houstonmethodist.org

Positioning and Anesthesia Concerns

- Left lateral decubitus position
  - The patient is taken to the operating room and placed on the operative table in the supine position.
  - After general anesthesia administration and double-lumen intubation, the Foley catheter is placed. If there is a concern for airway involvement, typically, patient has preoperative flexible bronchoscopy and endoscopic ultrasound with single-lumen tube to assess for resectability.
  - If a central line is necessary, it is typically placed on the right side.
  - The patient is then placed on the left lateral decubitus position with the right side up. The right chest is prepped for the procedure.
- Supine
  - After completion of the right chest portion of the procedure, the patient is placed in a supine position. The head is tilted to the right side with shoulder roll placed to expose the left neck. The patient's left neck, chest, and abdomen are prepped for the procedure.

Endoscopy with Fluoroscopy

- Endoscopy is performed with C-arm fluoroscopy. This helps to determine the location of the tumor in relation to the surgical anatomy. The endoscope is placed at the proximal part of the tumor, and a fluoroscope is performed to identify the location of the tumor in relation to the carina.

Right Chest: Port Placement

- Prep and drape the right chest in the usual standard fashion.

M. P. Kim (ed.), *Atlas of Minimally Invasive and Robotic Esophagectomy*, https://doi.org/10.1007/978-3-030-55669-3_5

- Make a 1 cm incision in the seventh intercostal space at the scapula tip. Using Xcel 5-mm trocar with a 5 mm camera, check the chest cavity using direct vision and insufflate the chest to 10 mmHg.
- Place a 12 mm robot port anterior in the seventh intercostal space right above the diaphragm (Arm 4) (Video 5.1) and another 8 mm robot port in the seventh intercostal space about 1/3 posteriorly from the 12 mm robot port when an imaginary line is drawn to the 5 mm port (Arm 3). Convert the first port to robot 8 mm port (Arm 1). Next, 8 mm robot port is placed in the 9th intercostal space along the scapula tip (Arm 2). Finally, a 12 mm Xcel or, if available, 12 mm AirSeal port is placed in the 4th intercostal space along the

scapula tip (Fig. 5.1a) (*this port is not necessary as you gain experience; Fig. 5.1b).

Docking the Robot

- Dock the robot.
- The green target is placed on the camera port (C). The arm is rotated around the camera port target to get the arm parallel to the ports in the seventh intercostal space.
- Arms are placed on the port.
- Arms are placed between "L" and "E" of the word FLEX on the arm (Fig. 5.2a).

Fig. 5.1 Photo of port placement with AirSeal port (**a**) or without AirSeal port (**b**)

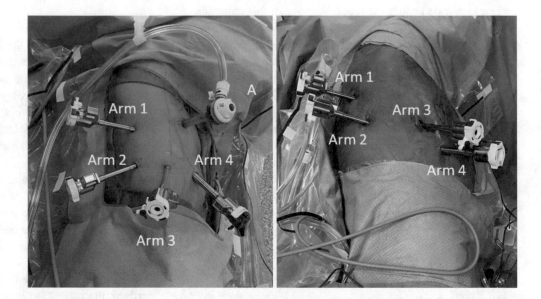

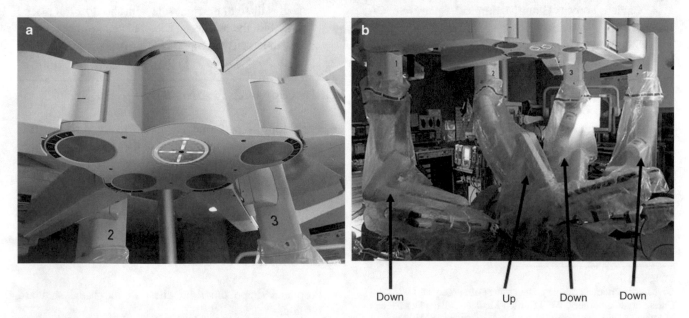

Fig. 5.2 Docking the robot. Photo of arms between the letter "L" and "E" of word "FLEX" (**a**). Arms are docked on the ports with Arms 1, 3, and 4 with patient clearance all the way down or extended and Arm 2 with patient clearance all the way up (**b**)

- Three arms that are in the 7th intercostal space (Arm 1, Arm 3, Arm 4), the patient clearance button is pressed to completely extend the arms.
- For Arm 2, the patient clearance button is pressed to completely collapse the arm (Fig. 5.2b).
- Two rolled Raytec is placed through the 12 mm port.
- A tip-up instrument is placed in the Arm1 port.
- A Cadiere is placed in the Arm 2 port.
- A vessel sealer is placed in the Arm 4 port.

Mobilization of Esophagus

- Use rolled Raytec to retract the lung anteriorly and hold the lung in place with a tip-up instrument from Arm 1 port.

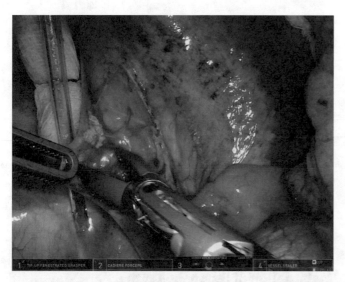

Fig. 5.3 Photo of dissection of the esophagus at the level of the inferior pulmonary vein

- Divide the pleura overlying the esophagus anteriorly and posteriorly all the way up to the azygous vein.
- Mobilize the azygous vein and divide using the robot vascular stapler.
- Divide the pleura overlying the esophagus anteriorly and posteriorly all the way up to the thoracic inlet.
- Dissect at the level of the inferior pulmonary vein around the esophagus (Fig. 5.3), and place a Penrose around it. Suture it with 3-0 silk.
- Pull the Penrose out through the Arm 2 port, and secure it on the drape forming a tension on the esophagus (Fig. 5.4). Place the Arm 2 port back, and place Cadiere grasper.
- Dissect the esophagus from the surrounding area. Ensure to keep the lymph nodes with the esophagus. Dissect close to the esophagus at the level of the left main bronchus. Dissect the esophagus away from the surrounding structures using the vessel sealer to the level of the thoracic inlet (Fig. 5.5).
- Place another Penrose around the esophagus, and suture it together with 3-0 silk. Place this Penrose in the thoracic inlet.
- Release the Penrose that was pulled out through the Arm 2 port, and place it above the diaphragm.

Mediastinal Lymph Node Dissection

- Remove station 7 and 9 lymph node. Use fenestrated curved bipolar in the Arm 4 port for dissection. Lymph nodes can be removed by placing a finger tip of a glove through the Arm 1 port, and the lymph node placed in the finger tip of a glove and it is sent to pathology.

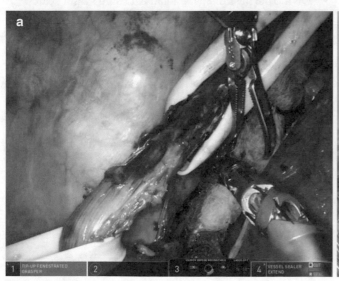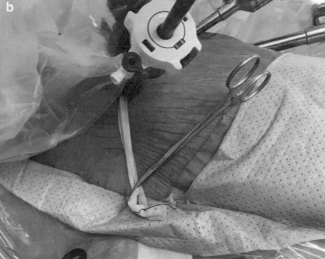

Fig. 5.4 Photo of two Penrose around the esophagus (**a**). The lower Penrose is pulled through the Arm 2 port and secured on the drape (**b**)

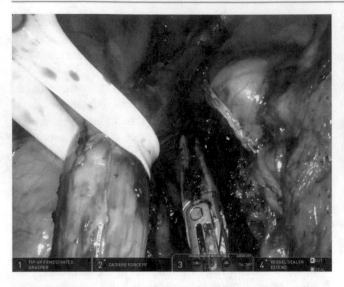

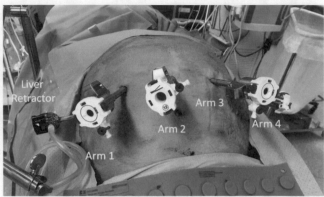

Fig. 5.6 Photo of abdominal port placement. The liver retractor is placed through the 5 mm lateral port. Arm 1 port or instrument port, Arm 2 or camera port, Arm 3 port or another instrument port, and Arm 4 port or last instrument port are visualized

Fig. 5.5 Photo of upper Penrose being held up to assist with dissection of the esophagus to the thoracic inlet

- Place a 5 mm Xcel port in the right upper quadrant below the liver edge. Place a liver retractor, and lift the left side of the liver to expose the gastroesophageal junction.
- Place the patient in reverse Trendelenburg about 30 degrees.

Closing the Right Chest

- Remove all instruments and undock the robot.
- Remove the rolled Raytec.
- Remove the ports.
- Place a 28 French chest tube through the camera port, and secure it with 0 silk.
- Close the incisions with 3-0 Vicryl in the subdermal layer and 4-0 Monocryl on the skin.

Docking the Robot (Fig. 5.7)

- Place the 30-degree camera in the port. Use the target function and set the robot arms.
- Dock the robot arms on the ports.
- Place Cadiere in Arm 1 and Arm 4 port and place vessel sealer in the Arm 3 port.

Abdomen: Port Placement (Fig. 5.6)

- Place the patient in a supine position with neck turned to the right side.
- Prep and drape patient's left neck, chest, and abdomen in usual standard fashion.
- Measure 12–13 cm from the xiphoid process toward the umbilicus in the midline, and mark this point. Measure 8 cm perpendicularly toward the left side, and mark it at this point. Place an Xcel 5 mm optical trocar using a 5 mm 0-degree camera, and enter the abdomen. Insufflate the abdomen to 15 mmHg.
- Place 12 mm robot port (Arm 2) at the midline about 12–13 cm from xiphoid process.
- Place 8 mm robot port (Arm 1) 8 cm from the midline port to the right side of patient perpendicular to the midline port. Place 8 mm robot port (Arm 4) about 8 cm lateral to the 5 mm Xcel port. Exchange 5 mm Xcel trocar to 8 mm robot port (Arm 3).

Mobilization of Esophagus at the Gastroesophageal Junction

- Divide the gastrohepatic ligament using vessel sealer.
- Mobilize the esophagus away from the right crus, diaphragm, and left crus.
- Dissect into the mediastinum and pull the Penrose into the abdomen (Fig. 5.8).
- Divide the right crus to widen the opening using the vessel sealer if the patient does not have a hiatal hernia.

Mobilization of the Stomach

- Using the Cadiere grasper through Arm 4 port, hold the mid stomach, and move the stomach toward the head to help visualize the greater curvature of the stomach and the greater omentum.

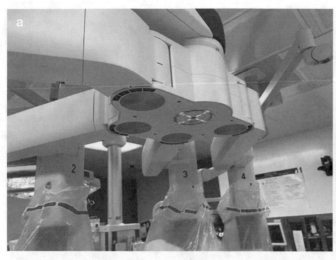 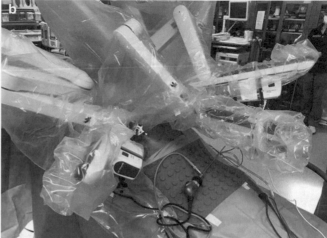

Fig. 5.7 Photo of FLEX joint (**a**) and the arms (**b**) docked to the port

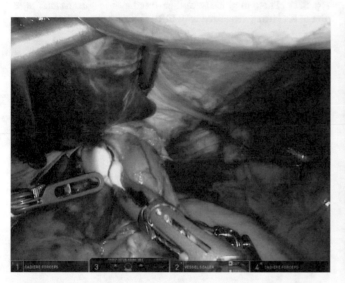 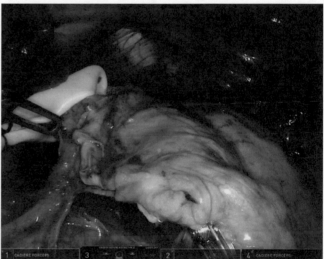

Fig. 5.8 Photo of dissection of the gastroesophageal junction and identification of the Penrose drain

Fig. 5.9 Photo of the left gastric artery

- Visualize the right and left gastroepiploic artery. Divide the omentum about 3 cm away from the gastroepiploic artery to enter the lesser curve. Use this entry point to divide the greater omentum and mobilize the greater curve of the stomach. Preserve as much of the gastroepiploic artery.
- Divide the short gastric artery.
- Divide the omentum preserving the right gastroepiploic artery to the pylorus
- Using the Cadiere grasper through Arm 4 port, lift the posterior stomach. Divide the avascular attachment from the posterior portion of the stomach to the pancreas until the left gastric artery can be visualized.
- Next, position the stomach so that the lesser curve is visualized. Extend the gastrohepatic ligament division to the stomach, preserving about four veins from the pylorus. Divide the vessels away from this portion of the stomach.

- Place the camera in the Arm 3 port. Place the robot vascular stapler in Arm 2 port, and divide the left gastric artery (Fig. 5.9).

Creation of Gastric Conduit (Fig. 5.10)

- Place robot blue load stapler at the Arm 2 port, and create the gastric conduit. The first staple line should be aimed toward the greater curvature of the stomach to create a conduit that is 3–4 cm in width. The rest of the stapler should be fired in parallel to the greater curvature of the stomach to create the gastric conduit.
- Mark the anterior portion of the gastric conduit with a marker to preserve orientation.
- Remove the Penrose.

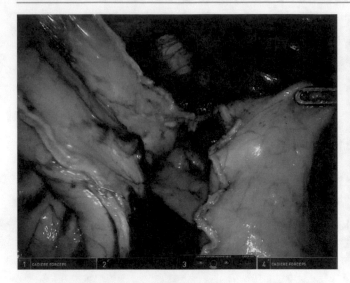

Fig. 5.10 Photo of gastric conduit divided from the specimen

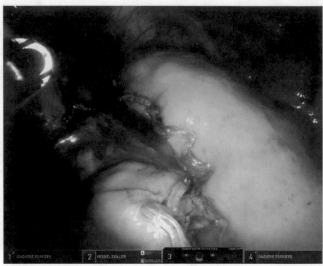

Fig. 5.11 Photo of globally well-perfused gastric conduit after injection of ICG being visualized with FIREFLY function on the robot

- Inject 3 cc of ICG, and turn on the FIREFLY function to visualize the perfusion of the gastric conduit. Determine if there is globally well-perfused conduit vs. demarcation. If there is a demarcation, mark it with a 3-0 silk suture (Fig. 5.11).
- Suture the tip of the conduit to the tip of the specimen where the gastric conduit was created using 2-0 Ethibond suture × 2.

Botox Injection to the Pylorus

- Inject 100 units of Botox diluted in 5 cc of NS in the pylorus at three different sites.

Undocking the Robot

- Remove instruments and undock the robot.
- Leave the ports and desufflate the abdomen.

Left Neck Dissection

- Make an incision in the left neck over the anterior portion of the sternocleidomastoid muscle about 2 cm from the sternal notch about 6 cm in length.
- Divide the platysma muscle layer.
- Mobilize the anterior portion of the sternocleidomastoid muscle.
- Divide the omohyoid muscle.
- Bluntly dissect down to the esophagus. Identify the Penrose and pull it up through the opening. Ensure not to put traction of recurrent laryngeal nerve.

Delivering the Specimen and the Conduit

- Insufflate the abdomen.
- Slowly pull the esophagus through the left neck while delivering the gastric conduit through the hiatus.
- Cut the suture between the specimen and the conduit in the neck.
- Remove the Penrose.
- Divide the esophagus at least 5 cm above the tumor but with adequate length of the esophagus for anastomosis.
- Send proximal margin for frozen section consultation to ensure there is no cancer at the margin.

Anastomosis: Modified Orringer (Fig. 5.12)

- Make an incision on the gastric conduit about 3 cm from the tip and suture that area to the esophagus.
- Place EndoGIA purple load stapler in the gastric conduit and the esophagus and fire the stapler.
- Close the opening between the esophagus and gastric conduit with 3-0 Vicryl in an interrupted fashion.
- Perform EGD to ensure that there is no leak at the anastomosis with a bubble test.
- Place the anastomosis in the neck/mediastinum.
- Place Penrose by the anastomosis and secure it with 3-0 silk on the skin.
- Close the incision with 3-0 Vicryl in interrupted fashion for the platysma layer. We then closed the skin with 4-0 Monocryl in running fashion.
- Place NG tube about 50 cm from the nose.

Fig. 5.12 Illustration of the anastomosis with gastric conduit and esophagus being anastomosed (**a**). Photo of left neck after the anastomosis (**b**)

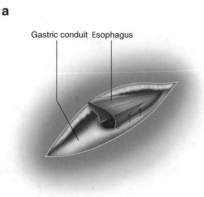

Gastric conduit Esophagus

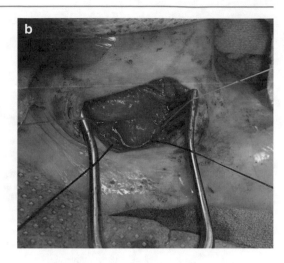

Jejunostomy Tube Placement

- Please see Chap. 8.

Closure of Abdomen

- Remove liver retractor and ports.
- Close the skin with 4-0 Monocryl.

Postoperative Care Consideration

- The patient is admitted to ICU after surgery.
- The head of bed is kept at 60 degrees at all time.
- The tube feed through the J-tube is started on postoperative day 1.
- The patient is transferred to the floor on postoperative day 1.
- The patient's NGT is typically removed day 2–3 after surgery.

- The patient's chest tube is removed on day 4 after surgery.
- The patient is typically discharged home on day 5–6 once patient is tolerating goal tube feeds. Penrose is removed prior to discharge.
- The patient returns to clinic about 2 weeks after surgery after esophagogram. If there is no signs of leak on esophagogram, patient's diet is advanced.

Suggested Reading

Patel S, Petrov R, Abbas A, Bakhos C. Robotic-assisted McKeown esophagectomy. J Vis Surg. 2019;5 https://doi.org/10.21037/jovs.2019.03.14. Epub 2019/08/21. PubMed PMID: 31428568; PMCID: PMC6698579.

Zhang H, Chen L, Wang Z, Zheng Y, Geng Y, Wang F, Liu D, He A, Ma L, Yuan Y, Wang Y. The learning curve for robotic Mckeown esophagectomy in patients with esophageal cancer. Ann Thorac Surg. 2018;105(4):1024–30. Epub 2017/12/31. PubMed PMID: 29288659. https://doi.org/10.1016/j.athoracsur.2017.11.058.

Techniques of the Chest Anastomosis

6

Edward Y. Chan

Introduction

Minimally invasive esophagectomy is most frequently performed via a transthoracic, transhiatal, or three-hole approach. While the definitions of "minimally invasive esophagectomy" vary widely, most would consider the term to signify both a laparoscopic or robot-assisted laparoscopic abdominal approach combined with a thoracoscopic or robot-assisted thoracoscopic chest approach. Our preferred technique is a minimally invasive robot-assisted laparoscopic and thoracoscopic Ivor Lewis esophagectomy. In this chapter, we will present step by step EEA anastomosis in the chest and highlight other commonly performed strategies.

Robot-Assisted EEA Stapled Anastomosis

Equipment

- Alexis GelPort (Applied Medical, Rancho Santa Margarita, CA)
- EEA 28 mm stapler with 3.5 mm staples (Medtronics, Minneapolis, MN)
- Xi Robot
  - Cadiere Forceps (Intuitive Surgical, Sunnyvale, CA)
  - Tip-Up Fenestrated Grasper (Intuitive Surgical, Sunnyvale, CA)
  - Mega SutureCut Needle Driver (Intuitive Surgical, Sunnyvale, CA)

Electronic supplementary material The online version of this chapter (https://doi.org/10.1007/978-3-030-55669-3_6) contains supplementary material, which is available to authorized users.

E. Y. Chan (✉)
Department of Surgery and Cardiothoracic Surgery, Weill Cornell Medical College, New York, NY, USA

Division of Thoracic Surgery, Department of Surgery, Houston Methodist Hospital, Houston, TX, USA
e-mail: eychan@houstonmethodist.org

- Long Bipolar Grasper (Intuitive Surgical, Sunnyvale, CA)
- Vessel sealer (Intuitive Surgical, Sunnyvale, CA)
- EndoWrist Stapler (Intuitive Surgical, Sunnyvale, CA)

Patient Position

- Left lateral decubitus position

Port Placement

- In order to optimize visualization and maximize working space, use five incisions in the right chest, including two 8-mm robotic ports, one 12-mm robotic port, one 12-mm AirSeal port, and a 3-cm incision with a Alexis GelPort wound protector through which we place a third 8-mm robotic port and which we also use for extraction of the specimen.
- Our incisions are arranged in a "five-on-a-dice" orientation, which we have previously described [1], that allows for a reproducible alignment which can be consistently applied to most robotic surgeries.
- The AirSeal port is placed in the 5th interspace in the midaxillary line, 8-mm ports are placed in the 7th interspace in the posterior axillary line and under the scapula tip, the 12-mm port is placed in the midaxillary line, and the GelPort is placed in 9th interspace posterior to the posterior axillary line.

Mobilization of the Esophagus

- Open the parietal pleura inferiorly overlying the esophagus and locate the Penrose drain around the intra-abdominal esophagus previously mobilized during the abdominal portion (Fig. 6.1) (Video 6.1).

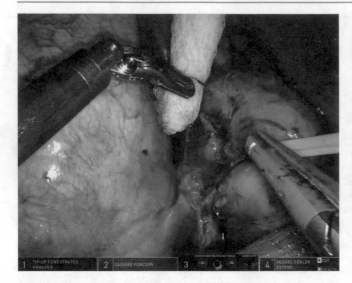

Fig. 6.1 Division of parietal pleura to identify the Penrose that was placed in the abdomen

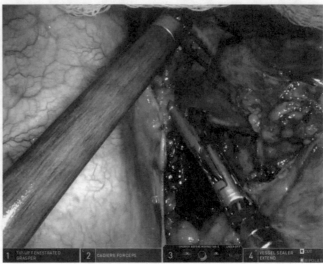

Fig. 6.2 Mobilization of the esophagus

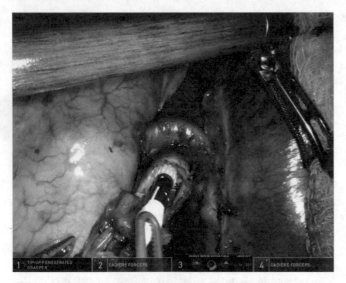

Fig. 6.3 EEA stapler anvil being inserted into partially divided esophagus

- Using the Penrose drain for retraction, mobilize the esophagus circumferentially to the level of the azygos vein. Divide the azygos with a vascular stapler.
- TIP: Improved retraction may be achieved by pulling the Penrose out of the chest outside of the GelPort and clamping it to the drape, thus freeing a robotic arm for dissection or retraction.
- TIP: Dissection should be performed close to the esophagus particularly at the level of carina to minimize the risk of injury to the airway. Special care must be taken to avoid injury to the membranous airway of the left mainstem bronchus. The subcarinal lymph node packet may be dissected free separately from the esophagus (Fig. 6.2)

EEA Anastomosis

- Partially divide the esophagus to allow for insertion of the EEA stapler anvil. We prefer a 28-mm EEA stapler with 3.5 mm staples. The level of division should be determined by the proximal extent of the tumor to ensure an adequate 5 cm margin (Fig. 6.3).
- NOTE: An anastomosis just distal to the azygos should provide adequate margin for most distal esophageal tumors. Division of the azygos will nevertheless minimize the risk of anastomotic restriction.
- Complete division of the esophagus with a robotic stapler, closing the distal end of the proximal esophagus with the anvil inside. Divide the proximal margin of esophagus, and send it for frozen section to ensure adequate margins (Fig. 6.4).
- Use bipolar and Bovie on the staple line. Pull the anvil out of the proximal esophagus adjacent to the staple line (Fig. 6.5). Place a purse-string suture around the anvil to help ensure that the mucosa is entirely contained within the subsequent EEA staple line (Fig. 6.6).
- Specimen, gastric conduit with omentum is brought into the chest through the gastroesophageal junction (Fig. 6.7).
- NOTE: We prefer to harvest a generous tongue of omentum adjacent to the gastric conduit during the abdominal portion of the operation. Transfer the omentum at this point into the chest with the conduit. We place the omentum in the mediastinum medial to the anastomosis to minimize the chance of mediastinitis in the event of an anastomotic leak.
- Place the gastric conduit next to the anvil and mark the area on the greater curvature of the gastric conduit where there is no tension and it sits next to the anvil.

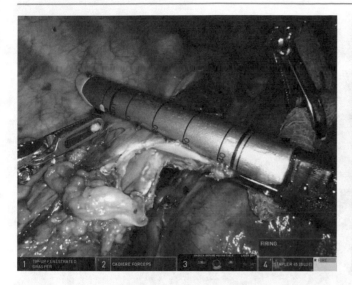

Fig. 6.4 Complete division of esophagus with anvil inside of the esophagus

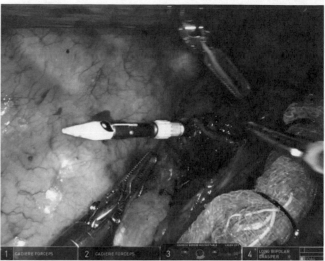

Fig. 6.5 Anvil through the esophageal staple line

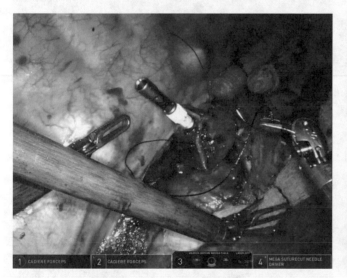

Fig. 6.6 Purse-string suture around the anvil

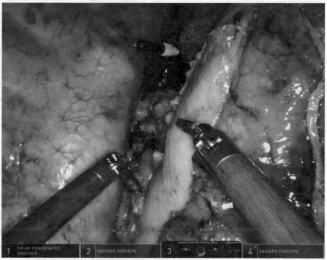

Fig. 6.7 Specimen and gastric conduit in the chest

- Eviscerate the tip of the esophagus through the GelPort and place a 0 silk stay suture. Place a hemostat on the silk and push the esophagus back into the chest.
- Eviscerate the tip of the specimen (Fig. 6.8) through the GelPort. Make an incision next to the stapler line at the tip of the specimen using the cautery so that EEA stapler can be easily placed in the specimen. Place four traction stitches evenly spaced around the opening, and then replace the specimen.
- Place the EEA stapler in the chest and place it in the tip of the specimen with help of four traction stitches (Fig. 6.9).
- Marry the ends of the EEA stapler, taking care to have the spike of the EEA handle protrude from the end of the gastric conduit where the anastomosis will lie (Fig. 6.10). Verify that the EEA donuts are complete

rings and send the donuts for frozen section to check for negative margins.
- TIP: Use the FIREFLY lens of the robot after injection of 3 cc of ICG followed by 10 cc of NS via IV to verify viability of the gastric conduit at the location of the planned anastomosis.
- Use a handheld EndoGIA stapler with purple load to complete the division of the distal esophagus/proximal stomach specimen from the gastric conduit.
- Place reinforcing simple interrupted stitches with 3-0 silk as needed in the anastomosis.
- An air leak test may be performed with endoscopic assessment of the anastomosis and conduit. Place a nasogastric tube under endoscopic visualization at this time. The omental flap may also be sutured in place at this time.

Fig. 6.8 Gastric conduit is
created in the abdomen with
stapler. The gastric conduit is
left on the specimen. The tip
of the specimen that is
illustrated is the area that is
eviscerated to place stay
sutures for the EEA stapler

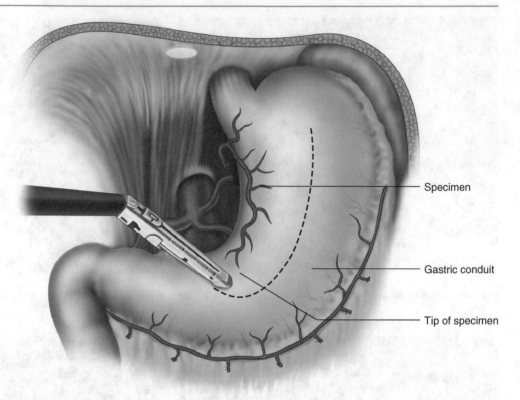

Specimen

Gastric conduit

Tip of specimen

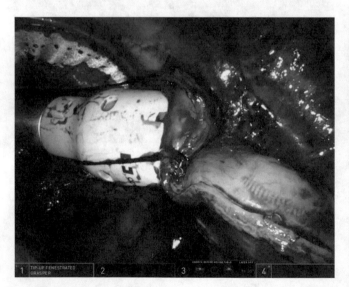

Fig. 6.9 EEA stapler going into the tip of the specimen

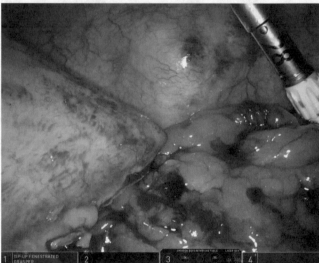

Fig. 6.10 Spike of EEA stapler coming through the gastric conduit

Variations on the EEA Anastomosis

Special Equipment

- Endo Stitch (Medtronic, Minneapolis, MN)
- Endoloop (Ethicon, Johnson & Johnson, New Brunswick, NJ)
- OrVil (Medtronic, Minneapolis, MN)

Purse String

- Minimally invasive technique: EEA anvil can be placed in the esophagus, and it can be secured with 2-0 Ethibond Endo Stitch. A purse string is created to get the esophagus around the anvil. Next, a baseball suture is created to get the end of the esophagus flush against the anvil. Make sure stitch takes a bite of the esophageal mucosa.
- TIP: Endoloop ligature can be used in addition to the sutures to ensure that the esophagus is snug against the anvil.
- Robot-assisted technique: 2-0 Ethibond can be used to place the purse-string suture followed by baseball suture to secure the esophagus around the anvil.

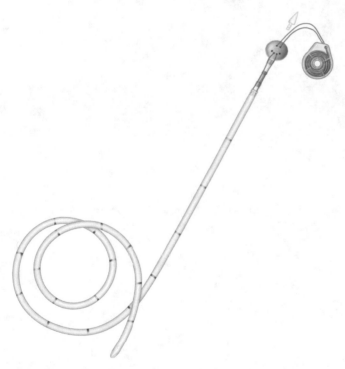

Fig. 6.11 Anvil of DST Series EEA OrVil attached to tube

OrVil

- Esophagus is stapled with either EndoGIA purple load stapler with thoracoscopic technique or robot blue load stapler.
- The tube attached to the 25 mm OrVil anvil (Fig. 6.11) is placed from the mouth to the tip of the stapled esophagus. Make sure to hold on to the string that is attached to the anvil when advancing the tube in the mouth. Either cautery or bipolar is used to get the tube through the tip of the esophagus.
- The string that is holding the anvil to the tube is cut and the tube is removed. The string from the mouth can also be removed.
- Marry it to the 25 mm EEA stapler in the gastric conduit to create the anastomosis.

Other Anastomotic Technique

- The majority of the surgeons who are performing robot-assisted Ivor Lewis Esophagectomy use an EEA anastomosis. Other options include a hand-sewn anastomosis and a linear stapled anastomosis. The two most common linear stapled anastomosis are the modified Collard (Chap. 4) and the modified Orringer (Video 6.2)

References

1. Kim MP, Chan EY. "Five on a dice" port placement for robot-assisted thoracoscopic right upper lobectomy using robotic stapler. J Thorac Dis. 2017;9(12):5355–62.

Suggested Reading

Egberts JH, Biebl M, Perez DR, Mees ST, Grimminger PP, Muller-Stich BP, Stein H, Fuchs H, Bruns CJ, Hackert T, Lang H, Pratschke J, Izbicki J, Weitz J, Becker T. Robot-assisted oesophagectomy: recommendations towards a standardised Ivor Lewis procedure. J Gastrointest Surg. 2019;23(7):1485–92. https://doi.org/10.1007/s11605-019-04207-y. Epub 2019/04/03. PubMed PMID: 30937716.

Jaroszewski DE, Williams DG, Fleischer DE, Ross HJ, Romero Y, Harold KL. An early experience using the technique of transoral OrVil EEA stapler for minimally invasive transthoracic esophagectomy. Ann Thorac Surg. 2011;92(5):1862–9. https://doi.org/10.1016/j.athoracsur.2011.07.007. Epub 2011/09/29. PubMed PMID: 21945228.

Kernstine KH. Minimally invasive Ivor-Lewis esophagectomy: use of the OrVIL device for the EEA intrathoracic anastomosis. Innovations (Phila). 2009;4(6):297–8. https://doi.org/10.1097/IMI.0b013e3181c4f8d8. Epub 2009/11/01. PubMed PMID: 22437224.

Okusanya OT, Hess NR, Luketich JD, Sarkaria IS. Technique of robotic assisted minimally invasive esophagectomy (RAMIE). J Vis Surg. 2017;3:116. https://doi.org/10.21037/jovs.2017.06.09. Epub 2017/10/29. PubMed PMID: 29078676; PMCID: PMC5639003.

Okusanya OT, Sarkaria IS, Hess NR, Nason KS, Sanchez MV, Levy RM, Pennathur A, Luketich JD. Robotic assisted minimally invasive esophagectomy (RAMIE): the University of Pittsburgh Medical Center initial experience. Ann Cardiothorac Surg. 2017;6(2):179–85. https://doi.org/10.21037/acs.2017.03.12. Epub 2017/04/28. PubMed PMID: 28447008; PMCID: PMC5387149.

Wee JO, Bravo-Iniguez CE, Jaklitsch MT. Early experience of robot-assisted esophagectomy with circular end-to-end stapled anastomosis. Ann Thorac Surg. 2016;102(1):253–9. https://doi.org/10.1016/j.athoracsur.2016.02.050. Epub 2016/05/08. PubMed PMID: 27154153.

Ray Chihara

There are many types of anastomotic techniques that may be employed in the neck from the cervical esophagus to the gastric conduit. The type of technique used varies mostly based on surgeon experience and training; however, length of available esophagus or conduit may affect the type of anastomotic techniques possible for the patient. Therefore, understanding of available techniques is important. Detailed descriptions of techniques used for the neck gastroesophageal anastomosis is described.

Many techniques are available for performing the cervical esophagus to gastric conduit anastomosis in the neck. In most cases, any technique can be utilized; however, certain conditions may only allow select techniques to be used. A more proximal location of a tumor may result in a shorter cervical esophagus available for anastomosis. Prior reflux operation, smaller stomach, and longer thorax length may limit amount of gastric conduit available for a neck anastomosis potentially leading to inability to perform the gastroesophageal anastomosis in the neck. Ensuring appropriate length for the anastomosis is therefore paramount. Techniques including the end-to-end linear stapled, side-to-side linear stapled, circular stapled, and hand-sewn anastomoses in the completed form are shown (Fig. 7.1).

The neck dissection and delivery of the gastric conduit into the left neck are the starting point for a gastroesophageal neck anastomosis. A complete stapled gastric conduit is delivered into the neck for all but the circular stapled anastomosis where a partially stapled gastric conduit is delivered into the neck (Fig. 7.2).

End-to-End Linear Stapled Anastomosis (Collard Anastomosis)

- The gastric conduit and remnant esophagus delivered through the cervical incision is oriented end to end [1].
- Perform partial resection of the esophagus to remove any redundant esophagus (Fig. 7.3a).
- The tip of the gastric conduit is opened slightly away from the staple line (Fig. 7.3a).
- The open end of the gastric conduit with staple line to the right of the patient is lined up next to the open end of the esophagus ensuring there is no twisting of the conduit or esophagus.
- The conduit and remnant esophagus are longitudinally paired, and a 3-0 silk interrupted Lembert is used to maintain orientation.
- A linear stapler is then chosen for the anastomosis. Common choices are Endo GIA™ blue (without Tri-Staple) or purple load (with Tri-Staple) 60 mm and Echelon Flex™ ETS 60 mm stapler with gold load.
- A linear stapler is then placed into the lined-up end-to-end conduit and remnant esophagus (Fig. 7.3b).
- The stapler is then fired to create a common channel approximately 40–50 mm in length (Fig. 7.3c).
- The opening is then closed using absorbable suture, 3-0 Vicryl or 4-0 PDS, in running fashion followed by 3-0 silk interrupted Lembert sutures (Fig. 7.3d).
- Alternatively, the opening may be closed using the same linear stapler after placing several suspension sutures (Fig. 7.3c) [2].

R. Chihara (✉)
Department of Surgery and Cardiothoracic Surgery, Weill Cornell Medical College, New York, NY, USA

Division of Thoracic Surgery, Department of Surgery, Houston Methodist Hospital, Houston, TX, USA
e-mail: rchihara@houstonmethodist.org

Fig. 7.1 The completed
end-to-end linear stapled,
side-to-side linear stapled,
circular stapled, and
hand-sewn anastomoses are
shown

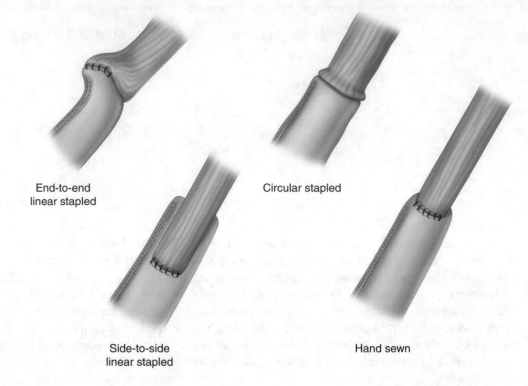

End-to-end
linear stapled

Circular stapled

Side-to-side
linear stapled

Hand sewn

Fig. 7.2 The starting point
for performing the neck
anastomosis is shown for in
the main image for the
end-to-end linear stapled,
side-to-side linear stapled,
and hand-sewn anastomoses.
The separate boxed image
shows the starting point for
the circular stapled
anastomosis

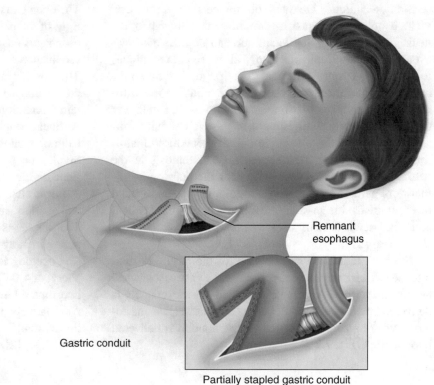

Remnant
esophagus

Gastric conduit

Partially stapled gastric conduit

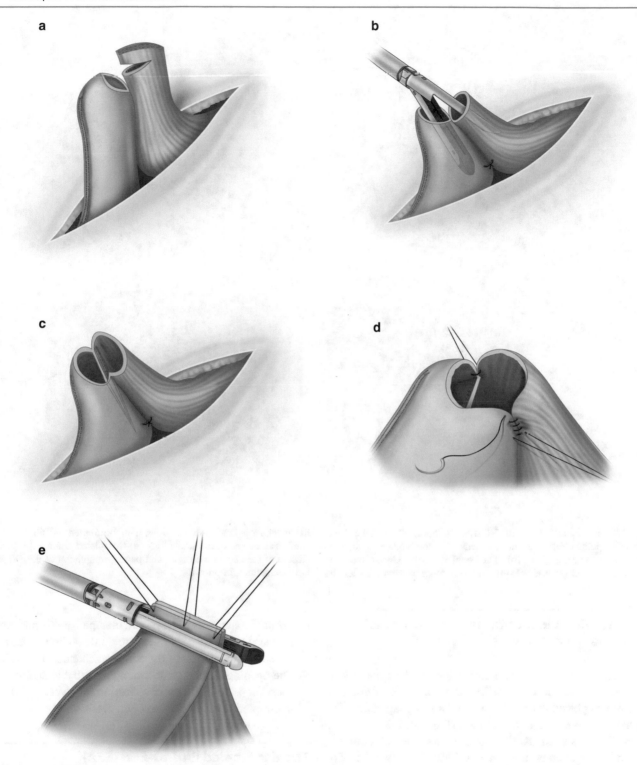

Fig. 7.3 (**a**) The gastric conduit with gastrostomy and esophagus with partial resection of redundant esophagus is shown. (**b**) A 3-0 silk Lembert stitch is placed at the base of the lined-up gastric conduit and esophagus, and the linear stapler is introduced into the gastrostomy and open esophagus. (**c**) The completed common channel is created after the stapler has been fired. (**d**) Corner silk 3-0 stay sutures are shown. Partially completed running 3-0 Vicryl closure of the common channel is shown. (**e**) Alternative closure of the common channel with a linear stapler is shown

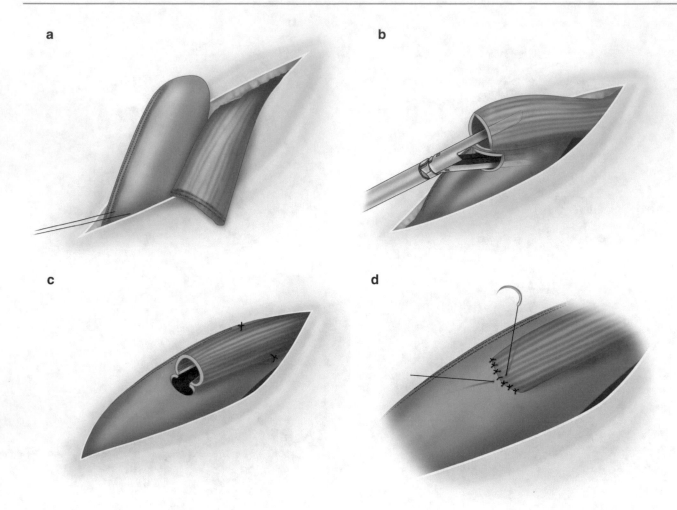

Fig. 7.4 (**a**) The retraction silk 3-0 stitch is shown allowing the stomach to be delivered further into the neck to accommodate the side-to-side linear anastomosis. (**b**) The stapler is introduced into the gastrostomy and open esophagus. (**c**) The common channel after the linear stapler is fired is shown along with interrupted 3-0 silk Lembert stitches at the end of the staple line. (**d**) Completed running 3-0 Vicryl closure of the common channel and partial completion of the 3-0 silk Lembert sutures are shown

Side-to-Side Linear Stapled Anastomosis (Orringer Anastomosis)

- The gastric conduit with staple line to the right side is brought into the cervical incision, and a retraction silk stitch is placed in conduit to allow for overlap of the remnant esophagus over the conduit (Fig. 7.4a) [3].
- A linear stapler is then chosen for the anastomosis. Common choices are Endo GIA™ blue (without Tri-Staple) or purple load (with Tri-Staple) 60 mm and Echelon Flex™ ETS 60 mm stapler with gold load.
- The remnant esophagus is lined up along with the gastric conduit, and site for gastrotomy is determined. The gastrotomy is performed, and the esophageal staple line or redundant esophagus is resected followed by placement of the linear stapler into the lined-up side-to-side gastric conduit and remnant esophagus (Fig. 7.4b).

- While the stapler is in place and clamped, a 3-0 silk stitch is placed at the corner of the staple line on both sides followed by completion of the common channel (Fig. 7.4c).
- The opening is then closed using absorbable suture, 3-0 Vicryl or 4-0 PDS, in running fashion followed by 3-0 silk interrupted Lembert sutures (Fig. 7.4d).

Circular Stapled End-to-End (EEA) Anastomosis Is Described

- The gastric conduit is oriented in the cervical incision with the partially completed conduit staple line to the right side. A stay suture is placed at the corner of the specimen side of the partially completed conduit followed by partially opening the specimen side staple line. Additional stay sutures are placed to allow retraction for the stapler (Fig. 7.5a).

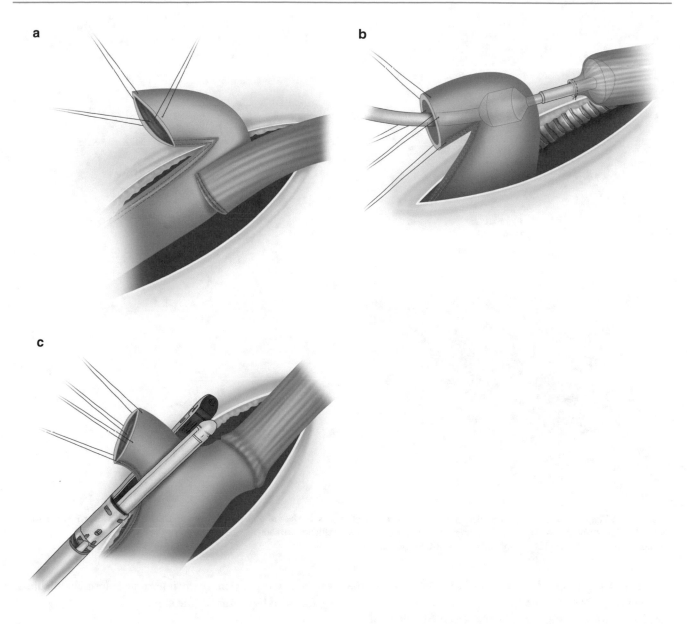

Fig. 7.5 (**a**) The opened staple line on the partially completed gastric conduit is shown with 0 silk retraction sutures in place. (**b**) The anvil with purse string in the esophagus and circular stapler through the partially completed gastric conduit with the stapler mated with the anvil is shown. (**c**) A linear stapler is shown completing the gastric conduit and resecting the remnant stomach used for the circular stapled anastomosis

- A circular stapler and load are then chosen. Common choices are EEA™ circular stapler with Tri-Staple™ 28 mm purple load, EEA™ circular stapler with DST Series™ 25–3.5 mm, or Ethicon circular stapler 25 mm or 29 mm. Generally, the largest anvil that can fit without injury to the esophagus is chosen.
- The anvil of the stapler is placed into the remnant esophagus, and purse string is made at the anastomosis (Fig. 7.5b).
- The circular stapler is placed into the gastric conduit, and a spot for the anastomosis is decided. The device trocar is extended through the gastric conduit and mated with the anvil, and the stapler is fired (Fig. 7.5c).

- The stapler is removed from gastric conduit and complete donuts are confirmed. The specimen side of the conduit is then stapled off using a linear stapler, e.g., EndoGIA™ purple load 60 mm stapler, completing the gastric conduit (Fig. 7.5d).

Hand-Sewn Anastomosis Techniques

- A location on the gastric conduit is chosen for creating the anastomosis, and the esophagus is positioned over the chosen site. Interrupted 3-0 silk esophageal muscle to seromuscular gastric conduit Lembert sutures are placed

a

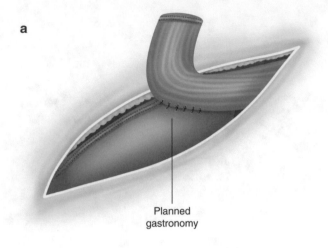

Planned
gastronomy

b

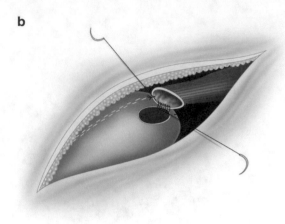

c

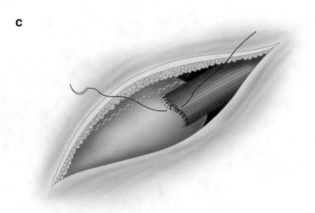

Fig. 7.6 (**a**) The back row 3-0 silk Lembert sutures are shown for the hand-sewn anastomosis. (**b**) The partially completed running 3-0 Vicryl anastomoses is shown. (**c**) The completed running 3-0 Vicryl anastomo- ses is shown, and partially completed 3-0 silk interrupted Lembert stitches are shown

between the posterior aspect of the esophagus and the planned gastrotomy site as the back row (Fig. 7.6a).

- The gastrotomy is then made followed by resection of any redundant esophagus. A running 3-0 Vicryl or 4-0 PDS suture through mucosa of the esophagus and gastric conduit approximating and inverting the mucosa with each travel (Fig. 7.6b).
- Once the running suture is completed, anterior 3-0 silk interrupted Lembert sutures are placed to complete the two-layer anastomosis (Fig. 7.6c). Alternatively, a single layer 3-0 Vicryl or 4-0 PDS running or interrupted technique could be used skipping the Lembert sutures.

Neck Incision Closure

- Completed anastomosis is oriented back into the neck.
- Place a Penrose drain into the mediastinum and orient to exit at the inferior aspect of the neck incision.

- Close the platysma with interrupted absorbable sutures followed by closure of the skin.

References

1. Collard JM, Romagnoli R, Goncette L, Otte JB, Kestens PJ. Terminalized semimechanical side-to-side suture technique for cervical esophagogastrostomy. Ann Thorac Surg. 1998;65(3):814–7. https://doi.org/10.1016/s0003-4975(97)01384-2. PubMed PMID: 9527220.
2. Tsuji T, Ojima T, Nakamori M, Nakamura M, Katsuda M, Hayata K, Kitadani J, Maruoka S, Shimokawa T, Yamaue H. Triangulating stapling vs functional end-to-end stapling for cervical esophagogastric anastomosis after esophagectomy for thoracic esophageal cancer: study protocol for a randomized controlled trial. Trials. 2019;20(1):83. https://doi.org/10.1186/s13063-019-3201-2. PubMed PMID: 30691515; PMCID: PMC6350379.
3. Orringer MB, Marshall B, Iannettoni MD. Eliminating the cervical esophagogastric anastomotic leak with a side-to-side stapled anastomosis. J Thorac Cardiovasc Surg. 2000;119(2):277–88. https://doi.org/10.1016/S0022-5223(00)70183-8. PubMed PMID: 10649203.

Robot-Assisted Jejunostomy Tube Placement

Min P. Kim

Introduction

Jejunostomy tube placement during esophagectomy allows for earlier enteric feeding, while the esophagogastric conduit anastomosis undergoes a healing process and strengthens over time. There are several complications that could arise from the placement of a jejunostomy tube. Two main concerns are bile leak onto the skin at the site of tube placement and clogging of the jejunostomy tube. We found that patients with smaller tubes tend to have less leaks around the tube but highly likely to clog, while bigger tubes tend not to have issues with clogging but high risk of developing a leak. The leak around the J-tube is very challenging problem. The technique presented in this chapter seems to provide low leak rate around the tube with low incidence of clogging of the tube (Video 8.1).

Equipment

J-tube

- 14 Fr MIC* jejunal feeding tube (Kimberly-Clark, Dallas, TX; Fig. 8.1)
- 16 Fr Argyle™* Pull-Apart Introducer Set (Medtronics, Minneapolis, MN; Fig. 8.2)

Xi Robot

- Cadiere Forceps × 2 (Intuitive Surgical, Inc, Sunnyvale, CA)

Electronic supplementary material The online version of this chapter (https://doi.org/10.1007/978-3-030-55669-3_8) contains supplementary material, which is available to authorized users.

M. P. Kim (✉)
Division of Thoracic Surgery, Department of Surgery and Cardiothoracic Surgery, Weill Cornell Medical College Department of Surgery, Houston Methodist Hospital, Houston, TX, USA
e-mail: mpkim@houstonmethodist.org

- Mega SutureCut™ Needle Driver (Intuitive Surgical, Inc, Sunnyvale, CA)

Positioning

- Supine

Port Placement

- Enter the abdomen in the right mid quadrant using 5 mm Xcel Optiview trocar (12 cm from the xyphoid process and 8 cm to the right side) if jejunostomy is performed independently to esophagectomy. Using laparoscopic technique, the rest of the ports are placed in the abdomen.
- Place 8 mm robot ports at right mid quadrant, right lower quadrant (midclavicular line below the level of the umbilicus), and left lower quadrant (midclavicular line below the level of the umbilicus) (Fig. 8.3).
- Place the jejunostomy tube in the left lower quadrant approximately 13–15 cm down from xyphoid process in the midline and 16 cm from that point to the left side of the abdomen above the level of the umbilicus. Mark the area of the J-tube on the skin.

Docking the Robot

- Xi Robot is positioned around the right lower quadrant port. A 30-degree camera is placed in the right lower quadrant port. Place Cadiere Forceps in the right mid-quadrant port and left lower quadrant port.

Jejunum

- Lift the colon toward the head to find the ligament of Treitz. We typically travel down the jejunum between

M. P. Kim (ed.), *Atlas of Minimally Invasive and Robotic Esophagectomy*, https://doi.org/10.1007/978-3-030-55669-3_8

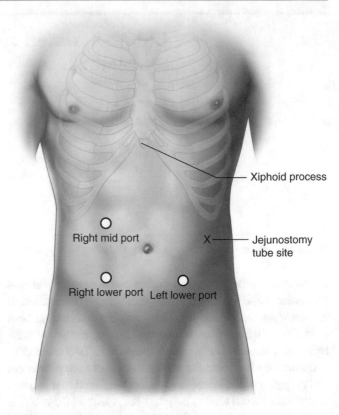

Fig. 8.3 Port placement

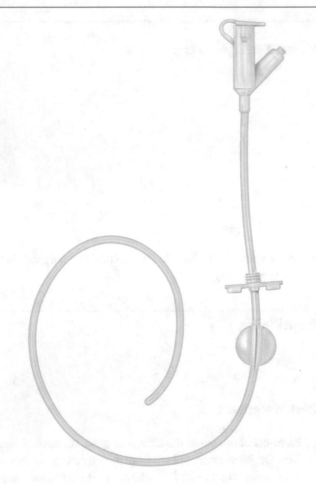

Fig. 8.1 MIC* jejunal feeding tube, 14 French

15 and 20 cm from the ligament of Treitz. This area is kept in view to ensure the correct placement in the jejunum.

- Bring 3-0 silk suture that is cut to 20 cm through the left lower quadrant port by bedside assistant to Cadiere Forceps in the surgeon's left arm.
- A Mega SutureCut™ Needle Driver is placed in the left lower quadrant port in the surgeon's right arm.
- A needle is placed from the jejunostomy site marked on the skin into the abdomen.
- Jejunum is sutured to the abdominal wall posterior to the needle placement for the jejunostomy site (Fig. 8.4).

Placement of Sutures

- Place two purse-string sutures on the jejunum with 3-0 silk in the area where the jejunostomy tube will be placed (Fig. 8.5).
- A 3-0 silk suture is placed from the left side of the jejunum to the abdominal wall on the left side of the needle on the screen.
- A 3-0 silk suture is placed from the right side of the jejunum to the abdominal wall on the right side of the needle on the screen.

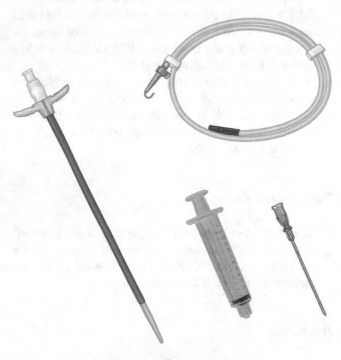

Fig. 8.2 16 Fr Argyl Pull-Apart Introducer Set

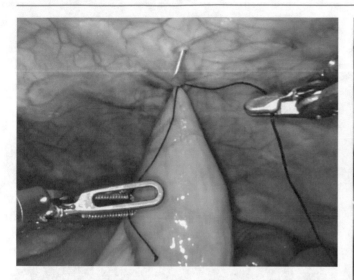

Fig. 8.4 Jejunum being sutured to abdominal wall

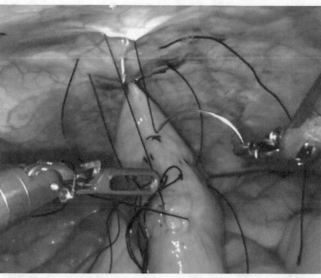

Fig. 8.6 Three sutures placed from the jejunum to the abdominal wall around the needle

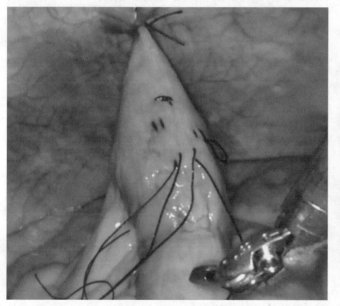

Fig. 8.5 Two purse-string sutures placed on the jejunum

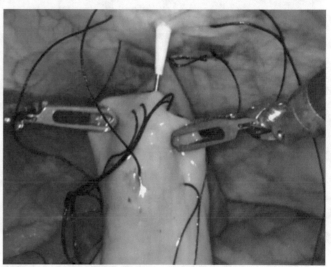

Fig. 8.7 16 Fr Pull-Apart Introducer with sheath advancing over a wire

- A 3-0 silk suture is placed from the distal end of the jejunum to the abdominal wall in the area that is nearest to the camera (Fig. 8.6).

Jejunostomy Tube

- Cadiere Forceps is placed in the left lower quadrant port. Using Cadiere Forceps, the jejunum is held at the suture that was placed on the left and right side and guided slowly to the needle while the assistant holds the needle in place. A 10 cc syringe with 5 cc of saline is placed on the needle. The needle is advanced slowly while the assistant draws back until there is air in the needle. Then the fluid is flushed into the jejunum.

- Next, the syringe is removed, and the wire is placed through the needle. Make sure the wire is in the jejunum going to the distal end of the jejunum.
- Needle is removed and 1.5 cm incision is made on the skin incorporating the wire.
- 16 Fr Argyle Pull-Apart sheath with the introducer is placed over the wire (Fig. 8.7), which slowly dilates the abdominal wall and enters the jejunum. Make sure to visualize the distal end of the introducer and let it advance slowly over the wire into the distal jejunum. Straighten out the distal jejunum so that the introducer with sheath enters the bowel unimpeded.
- Remove the wire and the introducer and leave the sheath in place.

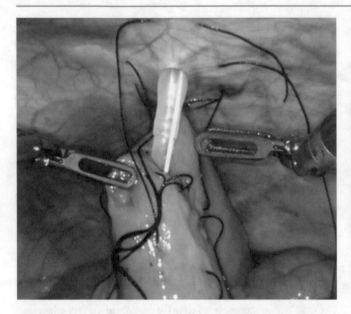

Fig. 8.8 The balloon part of jejunostomy tube being placed in the jejunum

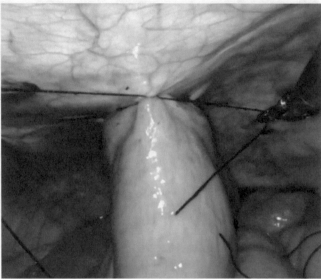

Fig. 8.10 Jejunum being tied to abdominal wall

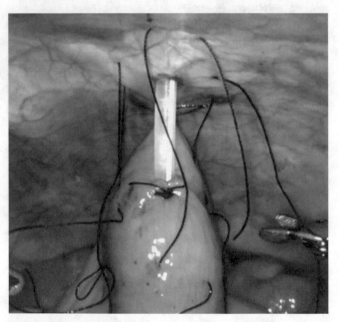

Fig. 8.9 Two purse strings tied around the jejunostomy tube

- Cut the 14 Fr Mic J-tube at the fold from the end to the balloon, and then wet the tube in sterile saline.
- Place the 14 Fr Mic J-tube in the sheath, and watch the distal end go into the jejunum.
- Once the balloon is at the skin, remove the sheath using the peel-away technique.
- Using the Cadiere Forceps, pull the balloon into the abdomen, and gently push it into the jejunum (Fig. 8.8). Advance it about 2 cm into the jejunum.
- Place 3 cc of water in the balloon and then pull the jejunostomy tube out to allow the balloon cusp to be right at the jejunum.

- Place Mega Suture Cut Needle Driver in the left lower quadrant port.
- Inner purse-string suture is tied followed by outer purse-string suture (Fig. 8.9). The jejunostomy tube is pulled out to allow apposition between the abdominal wall and the jejunum. Other three sutures are tied between the abdominal wall and the jejunum starting from screen right side of the jejunum, screen left side of the jejunum, and the distal suture (Fig. 8.10).
- The disk is advance toward the skin. A 2-0 nylon suture is loosely placed between the disk and the skin.

Closure of the Skin

- Robot is undocked.
- Ports are removed.
- Close the skin with 4-0 Monocryl.

Suggested Reading

Bakhos C, Patel S, Petrov R, Abbas A. Jejunostomy-technique and controversies. J Vis Surg. 2019:5. https://doi.org/10.21037/jovs.2019.03.15. Epub 2019/07/20. PubMed PMID: 31321215; PMCID: PMC6638548.

Siow SL, Mahendran HA, Wong CM, Milaksh NK, Nyunt M. Laparoscopic T-tube feeding jejunostomy as an adjunct to staging laparoscopy for upper gastrointestinal malignancies: the technique and review of outcomes. BMC Surg. 2017;17(1):25. https://doi.org/10.1186/s12893-017-0221-2. Epub 2017/03/23. PubMed PMID: 28320382; PMCID: PMC5359869.

Index

© Springer Nature Switzerland AG 2021
M. P. Kim (ed.), *Atlas of Minimally Invasive and Robotic Esophagectomy*, https://doi.org/10.1007/978-3-030-55669-3